Herbal Healing Secrets for Women

Safe, Natural Remedies for 40+ Women

Laurel Vukovic M.S.W.

PRENTICE HALL PRESS

Library of Congress Cataloging-in-Publication Data

Vukovic, Laurel.
    Herbal healing secrets for women / Laurel Vukovic.
        p. cm.
    Includes index.
    ISBN 0-7352-0102-1 (pbk.) — ISBN 0-13-012104-5 (cloth)
    1. Herbs—Therapeutic use.   2. Women—Health and hygiene.   I. Title.
RG129.H47 V85 1999
615.'321'082—dc21   99-056133
                                                             CIP

Acquisitions Editor: *Doug Corcoran*
Production Editor: *Eve Mossman*
Formatting/Interior Design: *Robyn Beckerman*

Printed in the United States of America

   10 9 8 7 6 5 4 3 2 1

This book is a reference work based on research by the author. The opinions expressed herein are not necessarily those of or endorsed by the publisher. The directions stated in this book are in no way to be considered as a substitute for consultation with a duly licensed doctor.

ISBN 0-7352-0102-1 (paper)   ISBN 0-13-012104-5 (case)

ATTENTION: CORPORATIONS AND SCHOOLS

Prentice Hall books are available at quantity discounts with bulk purchase for educational, business, or sales promotional use. For information, please write to: Prentice Hall Special Sales, 240 Frisch Court, Paramus, New Jersey 07652. Please supply: title of book, ISBN, quantity, how the book will be used, date needed.

PRENTICE HALL PRESS
Paramus, NJ 07652

On the World Wide Web at http://www.phdirect.com

Contents

Chapter 4

Be Cramp-Free   25

Chapter 5

Nip UTIs in the Bud   35

Chapter 6

Relieve Vaginal Infections Naturally   45

Chapter 7

Eliminate Fibroid Problems   53

Chapter 8

Healing Cervical Dysplasia   63

Chapter 9

Ease Fibrocystic Breast Discomfort   71

Chapter 10

Menopause: An Opportunity for Renewal   79

Chapter 11

Enhance Your Sexual Vitality   97

Chapter 12

Conquer Fatigue and Increase Your Energy   109

Chapter 13

Transform Stress and Anxiety 121

Chapter 14

Overcome Depression Naturally 139

Chapter 15

Sleep Well Every Night   149

Chapter 16

Keep Your Memory Sharp   159

Chapter 17

Control Hypoglycemia and Diabetes   167

Chapter 18

Relief for Varicose Veins 177

Chapter 19

Banish Migraine and Tension Headaches 185

Chapter 20

Hints for Healthy Digestion 193

Chapter 21

Maintain Strong Bones   203

Chapter 22

How to Keep Your Heart Healthy   215

Chapter 23

Avoid Developing Atherosclerosis   227

Chapter 24

How to Handle Hypertension 235

Chapter 25

Strengthen Your Immune System to Prevent Cancer 243

Chapter 26

How to Eat for Optimal Health 259

Chapter 27

Foreword

In the *Oxford English Dictionary*, "laurel" is an ancient evergreen tree whose foliage is used medicinally and is also the symbol of victory and distinction in the arts. I think our Laurel has distinguished herself exceedingly well in her book: *Herbal Healing Secrets for Women*. She has the gift of explaining complex health conditions clearly and her commonsense advice gives you every hope of being able to overcome them.

The book is very up-to-date, reflecting the latest research on herbal remedies and aromatherapy as well as such important topics as: homocysteine as a cause of heart disease; the problems with non-organic canola oil; and alerting us to the continued use of harsh chemicals in the cosmetic industry. The chapter on Natural Beauty supplies simple recipes for excellent alternatives. How much easier could a face mask be than mixing a tablespoon of avocado with some yogurt?

The chapter on Healthy Digestion gives vital information for determining food sensitivities through an elimination diet and offers an overview of a rotation diet. Since everyone is unique this is necessary information to help individualize the diet and eliminate problem foods.

Laurel also tackles the very tough topic of cancer and accurately demonstrates the primary cause as environmental toxins, chemicals, and radiation, which alter DNA and lead to a downward spiral of our immune system with impaired surveillance against mutating cells. It is terrifying but true that one in two people will be diagnosed with cancer in his or her lifetime and one in four will die from cancer. With these unbelievable statistics we not only have to make every effort to protect ourselves from toxic drugs and chemicals but we also have to take a stand for our environment. This is getting easier to do as we realize the power of the marketplace. The more we buy natural products, organic foods, and herbs as Laurel suggests, the more we visit alternative practitioners; the more we demand that research funds go into alternative treatments, the more we will steer big industry into "greener" pastures. At a time when leaders in the field of toxicology and environmental medicine are warning us to unburden ourselves from chemicals in our milieu, Laurel gives us crucial advice on detoxification and cleansing the body as well as natural herb substitutes for drugs and chemicals.

The chapter Cervical Dysplasia gives clear, concise, and effective solutions for a condition that, in its mild to moderate stages, is treated with a "wait-and-see" attitude. This can be very disconcerting and frightening for women who wish to heal the condition rather than getting more and more worried as the date of their next Pap test approaches. This "negative visualization" may even be detrimental, something that allopathic medicine is not attuned to; whereas Laurel gives simple advice including positive visualizations to put you in control of the situation. It is these types of proactive messages that are so important in this book.

Laurel also tackles fibroids, a condition that is most commonly treated with hormonal or surgical intervention. She presents many natural prescriptions for this condition that women can prepare, perhaps eliminating the need for drastic intervention. When the conventional approach is surgery, finding safe alternatives is a great relief.

Herbal Healing Secrets for Women is much more than just a book of herbal secrets, Laurel shares with us wonderfully lucid psychological descriptions of various life transitions, especially that of menopause, and offers gentle guidance and support for us to flourish during this special time. She also provides valuable information on diet and supplements as well as herbs that will ease this time of change. I love the term "mental-pause" for the all-too-common memory lapses that can be treated. And reminding women that sex gets better after menopause really helps to dispel some ridiculous myths. After all, why do you think all these men are rushing to Viagra? To keep up with their women!

I also appreciated the chapter on osteoporosis. As baby-boomers age, the incidence of osteoporosis is increasing. The medical approach is hormonal therapy or drug intervention. Over the years I have seen many drugs for osteoporosis touted as "cure-alls" and then banished when the side effects accumulate in the unsuspecting public. However, bone-building foods and herbs along with exercise are the most effective way to prevent osteoporosis. Native cultures don't develop osteoporosis but they also don't smoke, drink alcohol or eat a refined food diet. Laurel's advice is very important and practical as more and more of us realize we have to take matters into our own hands and change our lifestyle, utilizing diet to prevent or alleviate conditions such as osteoporosis.

Espousing herbal medicine however does not mean we abandon the best parts of Western medicine. That is what is so wonderful about the times in which we live. We can have it all. We can use safe, natural, inexpensive herbal alternatives for many common ailments. But if we need surgery or medications, they are also available and actually work better in a body that is strengthened by herbs. A healthy body is more able to deal with the side effects of medications and will even heal faster from surgery. And you can achieve a healthy body by simply following the commonsense advice in *Herbal Healing Secrets for Women*.

Carolyn F. A. Dean, M.D., N.D., C.C.N.

Introduction

You may have picked up this book because you have some concerns about your health, or perhaps you just want to know how to maintain your health and vitality at mid-life and beyond. You have already taken one of the most important steps toward healing, because ultimately, *you are your own best healer.* My purpose in writing this book is to provide you with the knowledge that will help you bring your body, mind, and spirit into balance, which allows for healing to occur. Over the years, I've learned that health and vitality, particularly after the age of 40, are primarily the result of how well we care for ourselves on a daily basis. For this, you need practical information that you can easily incorporate into your daily life.

Twenty-five years ago, when I was in college, my health seemed to be on a downward spiral. I was frequently battling a cold or flu, my energy was low, and I was plagued by allergies. I suffered from digestive upsets, hypoglycemia, and bouts of anxiety. Frustrated and worried, I consulted two doctors—one of whom told me (in response to my asking if he thought that changing my diet might help) that what I ate had absolutely nothing to do with my health. The second doctor ran a series of tests and found that my white blood cell count was abnormally and unexplainably low. When I asked him if he thought that my lowered immunity could be caused by emotional stress, he replied that my mind had no influence on my body. Fortunately, I didn't listen to either expert. My intuition told me that I needed to make some concrete changes in the way that I was caring for myself, and I began to explore nutrition, herbal healing, yoga, and meditation in an attempt to improve my health. Today, at age 46, I feel better than ever before in my life, and I feel confident that I have the knowledge to keep my body and mind in optimal health in the years to come.

My explorations into the world of healing have become more than a personal journey—they have become my life's work. My interest in the interrelationship of the mind and body led me to a master's degree in clinical social work with an emphasis in behavioral medicine. I worked for several years with women suffering from a wide range of physical problems—from PMS and insomnia to hypertension, diabetes, and cancer—helping them to make lifestyle changes to facilitate their healing. For the past ten years, I've been a writer and editor in the field of alternative medicine, and have been writing the Home Remedies column for *Natural Health* magazine for most of this time.

I love teaching and writing about self-care—sharing information about the ways that we can best care for ourselves, whether it's treating a bladder infection or preventing cancer. I am especially drawn to using herbs for healing. In my early twenties, just as I was beginning my exploration into the world of alternative healing, I serendipitously encountered an herbalist who was passing through town. I was on the verge of yet another bladder infection and stubbornly determined to not take antibiotics. She gave me a packet of herbs with instructions to brew a quart of tea, which I remember as incredibly bitter tasting. By the next morning, all symptoms of the infection had vanished, and I began to study and experiment with herbs in earnest. Since then, I have used herbs to successfully treat respiratory, bladder, and yeast infections, and I've seen herbs relieve hypertension, ease PMS and menopausal discomfort, and alleviate insomnia and anxiety. In fact, I can't really think of any condition—physical or emotional—where herbs can't be used to help to restore balance and promote healing. I am delighted at the renaissance taking place in herbal healing, and at the widespread interest in alternative health practices. The more we learn, and the more we share what we learn, the more empowered we become and the healthier we will all be.

Of course, in addition to using herbs for healing, building a good foundation of health practices is essential—eating well, exercising appropriately, and getting enough rest and relaxation. I also believe that for optimal health, we need to be comfortable within ourselves, to make peace with who we are and with others in our lives, and to learn to live with joy and gratitude. Health breakdowns most commonly occur after the age of 40, and for good reason. Years of less than optimal living habits have taken their toll, and many women become aware, perhaps for the first time, of signs of aging. This is an important time to pay exquisite attention to caring for yourself physically, emotionally, and spiritually. You will find your efforts greatly rewarded in terms of improved health and vitality and increased energy and joy in living.

It's important to recognize that while healing can occur remarkably quickly, it can also take many months to create a state of optimal well-being. Oftentimes, a natural approach to healing takes longer to produce results than conventional medical treatments such as drugs and surgery. But natural healing treatments are almost always more effective for treating chronic health problems, because instead of suppressing symptoms, you are addressing the root cause of the imbalance that allowed the disease to arise. This does not mean that you should turn your back on conventional medicine. In some circumstances, conventional medical treatments are appropriate, and even life-saving. However, in most cases, the natural approaches outlined in this book can be used along with conventional medicine, and will help to encourage your body's natural healing response. *If you have a serious medical condition such as cancer or heart disease, please work with a qualified health care professional to design a program of healing that is most appropriate for your condition.*

Whatever the state of your current health, you can take steps today to increase your physical, emotional, and spiritual well-being. I hope this book serves as a useful guide in your journey.

Chapter 1

Forty and Beyond: The Best Years of Your Life

At midlife, most women become aware, perhaps for the first time, of the changes that aging brings. Although none of us can stop growing older, we *can* slow down the aging process and enjoy vibrant health throughout the years of our lives. Midlife is a wonderful opportunity for pausing to evaluate where you are in your life and for envisioning how you would like to live in the years to come. These can be the most satisfying years of your life, because you have the opportunity to use the accumulated wisdom of your experiences to create your life as you want it to be.

In this book, you will find a wealth of information that can help you achieve lifelong health and vitality, from specific dietary and exercise advice to the use of herbs, aromatherapy, hydrotherapy, meditation, and visualization for healing. Central to the process of healing is self-understanding, because within you lies the knowledge that can guide you to

vibrant health. Your body and your psyche are continually com-
municating with you, but the messages are often muted because
of years of neglecting to listen. There are many ways that we
neglect ourselves, from overworking to overeating to allowing our
true desires to languish while we do what we think we "should"
be doing. One of the most powerful tools for healing is to learn to
listen carefully to the messages from your body and your psyche
and to honor yourself by taking the time to care for and nurture
yourself.

Living a healthful life is simple if you pay attention to your true
needs on a daily basis. The key is to cultivate awareness in the
moment. Are you tired? Give your body the rest that it needs. Are
you hungry? Nourish your body with satisfying, health-supportive
foods. Are you lonely? Reach out to someone who makes you feel
good. If you honor the subtle messages from your body and psyche, you can never get too far out of balance. While these may seem
like minor actions, it is the sum of the choices that you make on a
daily basis about how you live and care for yourself that determine
to a great extent how healthy and fulfilling your life will be in the
years that lie ahead of you. By adopting a health-supportive
lifestyle, you will feel great today, and you will also be building a
strong foundation for the decades of life that lie ahead.

Seven Keys to Aging Gracefully

1. **Have a purpose in life**. Women who enjoy long, fruitful lives
inevitably feel that they have a reason to live and a purpose that
they are meant to fulfill. This is different for every woman, because
each of us is unique. If you are not clear about your purpose in life,
begin by following what brings you joy and helps you to feel a part
of the whole. Know that it is never too late to begin doing what you
love and to cultivate listening more to your inner wisdom than to
external "shoulds."

2. **Accept and love yourself**. There is no one quite like you in
this world, nor is there likely to ever be again. Focus on appreciat-
ing the incredible gift of life that you have been blessed with, and
remind yourself daily that you have something special to offer to the

world. Loving and accepting yourself just as you are will free your energy to care for yourself in healthy ways.

3. **Learn to relax.** Learning to flow with life is essential for your well-being. No matter how healthfully you eat or how much you exercise, if you are chronically stressed your body and your mind will suffer, and your enjoyment of life will be dramatically diminished. Stress literally attacks your body and your brain by creating cell-destroying free radicals. Nourish a sense of physical and emotional calm through relaxation exercises, meditation, yoga, and other practices that you find balancing.

4. **Eat a diet of whole, natural foods.** Forget restrictive diets and focus instead on nourishing your body with a wide variety of delicious, fresh, whole, nutrient-dense foods. In addition, supplement your diet with extra vitamins, minerals, antioxidants, essential fatty acids, and other nutrients that are known to support health and longevity.

5. **Move your body daily.** Regular exercise strengthens your cardiovascular system, muscles, and bones, keeps you flexible, improves your circulation, brightens your mood, and helps you to maintain a healthful weight. Develop an appreciation and enjoyment of moving your body and experiment with different forms of exercise to find what is right for you.

6. **Avoid exposure to toxins.** Chemicals in foods and water, poisons in household and garden products, and environmental pollutants are major causes of free radicals, which damage your body's cells, cause degenerative disease, and accelerate the aging process. Make a deliberate effort to eliminate these harmful substances from your life.

7. **Cultivate joy.** Your mind plays a critical role in not only your mental health, but in your physical well-being. There are many ways to nourish a positive attitude, including consciously cultivating gratitude. The healthiest people are those who see challenges as opportunities for growth, instead of as obstacles. Feed your spirit daily in simple ways such as spending time in nature, being with family and friends whom you enjoy, and meditation. Discover what feels good to you, and do it every day.

How to Take Charge of Your Health

Following the seven steps outlined here will help you to stay healthy throughout your life. But all of us, at various times, encounter minor or major health concerns. Many of these health problems are chronic, nagging complaints such as headaches, fatigue, or vaginal infections, while others are serious degenerative diseases such as high blood pressure and diabetes that slowly erode health and vitality. Whatever the state of your current health, there are many positive steps that you can take to support your journey back to well-being. While conventional medicine tends to suppress the symptoms of disease, a natural approach to healing focuses on supporting your body's innate ability to heal itself. Many of the health problems that women experience at midlife and beyond can be safely and effectively treated with methods of natural healing that work in harmony with your body, including specific diet and exercise recommendations, massage and other bodywork techniques, aromatherapy, hydrotherapy, meditation and mind-body practices, and of course, the use of herbs for healing. Herbal healing is the primary focus of this book, but herbs are most powerful when used within the context of a holistic approach to health that takes into account your diet, lifestyle, the influence of your mind on your physical well-being, and a variety of other supportive healing therapies.

Herbal Secrets for Health and Longevity

There is a tremendous renaissance taking place in herbalism today because women (and men) are reclaiming personal responsibility for their health and well-being. There is something deeply satisfying about using herbs for healing. When I brew a cup of herbal tea, gather wild plants, make an herbal tincture or salve, or add nourishing herbs to a soup, I am aware of tapping into an ancient lineage of wisdom that has been passed down from the beginning of time, and I feel connected and grateful to all of the healers who have come before me. Herbal medicine is readily accessible to all of us—in fact, it is as close as the wild plants that grow in your own backyard.

Herbs are a particularly powerful healing ally for women. Traditionally, women have held the role of healers for their families and communities, and healing plants were their primary form of medicine. Through centuries of using the herbs that grew around them, women discovered which plants were effective for treating various health concerns, and they passed this wisdom down through the generations to create the body of knowledge that we draw from today for healing. Although Western medicine has become disconnected from the world of natural healing, many pharmaceutical drugs now in use were originally derived from plants, and the majority of the world's population still relies on herbs as their primary form of medicine.

In this book, you will discover potent, safe herbs for alleviating the symptoms of menstrual problems, menopausal difficulties, headaches, insomnia, and mood swings. You will learn how to use powerful health restorative herbs as part of a natural approach for treating serious degenerative conditions such as heart disease and diabetes. And you will learn the ancient secrets of herbs that have been revered for centuries as health, vitality, and longevity tonics. Each chapter of this book focuses on a specific health concern and offers a comprehensive approach to natural healing treatments that will help you to take charge of your health. Of course, if you suffer from any type of serious or chronic health condition, be sure to consult your health practitioner. Try to find someone who is open to natural healing modalities. The number of physicians and other health-care professionals who are incorporating alternative health practices into their treatments is steadily increasing as they discover the powerful healing potential of natural remedies.

Chapter 2

Herbs: Your Allies for Health and Healing

Knowing a few basic guidelines for selecting, storing, and preparing herbal remedies will help you to use herbs most effectively.

Guidelines for Selecting and Storing Herbs

DRIED HERBS

- Choose herbs that are brightly colored and fragrant; this will ensure more potent herbal preparations. Whenever possible, purchase organically grown herbs.

- Store each herb individually in a tightly lidded glass container. Pint- or quart-size canning jars are ideal.

- Heat and light destroy the healing properties of herbs. Store your herbs in a cool, dark, dry place, such as a cabinet, pantry, or closet.

- When properly stored, the dried leaves and flowers of herbs will retain their medicinal properties for approximately one year. Most roots and barks will retain their healing properties for about two years.

LIQUID EXTRACTS

- Liquid extracts (sometimes called tinctures) are made by steeping an herb in alcohol (such as grain alcohol or vodka) or vegetable glycerin. Alcohol best extracts the full range of medicinal properties of the herb and also acts as a preservative. Glycerin is less effective at extracting the healing constituents of the plant, but is a useful option for those who wish to avoid alcohol.

- You can evaporate most of the alcohol from a liquid extract by placing the dosage in a cup and pouring one-quarter cup of boiling water over it. Allow the water to cool for several minutes before drinking.

- Liquid extracts should be stored in a cool, dark, dry place. If stored properly, they will retain their potency for three to five years or even longer.

Making Herbal Preparations

Making your own herbal infusions, decoctions, and liquid extracts is quick and easy. Herbal infusions and decoctions are basically teas prepared in a specific way to maximize the healing properties of the herb. They are similar to teas in that the fresh or dried herb is steeped or simmered in hot water. Herbal infusions and decoctions are best prepared in glass, porcelain, earthenware, or enamel-coated steel pots. Stainless-steel pots are also fine, but avoid aluminum or nonstick cookware.

A typical dose of an herbal infusion or decoction is three to four cups a day. You can make a couple of quarts of infusion or decoction at a time and refrigerate it to use over two days. Gently warm the refrigerated tea before drinking. While most of the healing properties remain intact when made in this way, I prefer the flavor of freshly brewed herbs. Because it's often not convenient to brew one cup of infusion or decoction at a time, I find it easiest to prepare a quart of herbal infusion or decoction each morning and then to drink it throughout the day. If you are using the mixture within one day, it doesn't need to be refrigerated.

Herbal liquid extracts are made by steeping dried or fresh herbs in alcohol or vegetable glycerin for several weeks. Liquid extracts are convenient to use and make it easy to take herbs that are bitter or unpleasant tasting. A typical dose of an herbal extract is one-half teaspoon three times daily. Dilute the dosage in approximately one-quarter cup of warm water before taking.

How to Make an Herbal Infusion

If you've ever brewed a cup of herbal tea, you have made a simple herbal infusion. Infusions are made from the more delicate parts of the plant, such as the flowers, leaves, and seeds.

For a medicinal-strength infusion that retains all of the healing properties of the plant, use one to two teaspoons of dried herb for each cup of water. If you are using fresh herbs, increase the amount to one to two tablespoons. When using seeds such as fennel or anise, it's helpful to gently bruise them first in a mortar and pestle to release the essential oils.

Pour boiling water over the herb and immediately cover the container to keep the volatile essential oils from escaping in the steam. Steep for 10 to 15 minutes and strain. For a stronger infusion, allow the herb to steep until the liquid cools to room temperature before straining. If you are making an infusion to use in a bath or compress, increase the proportion to one tablespoon of dried herb to each cup of water.

How to Make an Herbal Decoction

A decoction extracts the medicinal properties from the tougher parts of the plant, typically the root and bark. To make a decoction, place the herb in cold water in a covered pot. Use one to two teaspoons of dried herb to each cup of water. Bring to a boil over medium heat, lower the heat as soon as it reaches a boil, and simmer, covered, for 15 minutes. Remove from heat, let steep for 15 minutes, and strain. For a stronger decoction, allow the herb to steep until the liquid cools to room temperature before straining. As with an infusion, if you are making a decoction to use in a bath or compress, increase the amount of herb to one tablespoon for each cup of water.

How to Make an Herbal Extract

To make an herbal extract, you will need dried or fresh herbs and enough vodka to cover the herbs by three inches. Buy cut or shredded dried herbs and grind them in a coffee grinder or blender until they are a coarse powder. Some roots and barks will not grind easily—don't worry about it, the medicinal properties will still be extracted. If you are using fresh herbs, chop them finely.

Pack the herbs loosely into a glass jar with a tight-fitting lid and add enough vodka to cover the herbs plus an additional three inches. Stir well, and cover. Keep in a warm, dark place for three weeks. Shake the jar daily to thoroughly mix the herbs and vodka. After three weeks, strain the liquid into a bowl through a colander or strainer lined with several layers of cheesecloth. Wring the herbs in the cheesecloth, squeezing them to extract any remaining liquid. Pour the liquid extract into dark glass bottles for storage.

Alcohol is the best liquid for extracting the medicinal properties of the herbs, but if you want to avoid alcohol, you can use vegetable glycerin. Follow the same steps as if you were making an alcohol extract, but replace the alcohol with a mixture of equal parts of vegetable glycerin and water. If you are using fresh herbs, use a mixture of three-quarters vegetable glycerin and one-quarter water to adjust for the water content of the fresh plant material.

How to Make an Herbal Salve

Herbal salves are also easy to make and provide the healing benefits of herbs in a concentrated form for using on the skin. Excellent herbs for making salves include *calendula* and *comfrey*, both of which have skin-healing properties.

To make an herbal salve in the traditional method, you first need to make an infused oil with the herb. Coarsely chop one-half cup of dried herb in a blender. Combine with one cup of olive oil in a wide-mouth glass jar with a lid and place in direct sunlight. The warmth of the sun helps to extract the medicinal properties of the herb. After one week, filter the oil through several layers of cheesecloth, straining out all herb particles. If any herb particles remain, strain through a coffee filter.

Combine one-half cup of herbal infused oil with two tablespoons of grated beeswax in a small, heavy saucepan. (Save the remaining oil for making more salve, or use as a massage oil.) Heat gently until the beeswax is melted. Pour the salve into a wide-mouth glass jar, let cool, and cover with a lid. When stored in a cool, dark place, an herbal-infused oil or salve will stay fresh for approximately one year.

Chapter 3

Say Goodbye
to PMS

I don't believe I've ever known a woman who hasn't suffered from premenstrual syndrome. By some estimates, as many as 90 percent of women in their reproductive years are affected to some degree by PMS. The symptoms may be mild enough to be merely noticeable, or so debilitating as to severely disrupt normal life. While it's normal to experience fluctuations in energy throughout the menstrual cycle, emotional and physical suffering are not inevitable. By paying attention to creating a healthful way of living and by using herbs and other natural remedies, you can say goodbye to PMS.

A PMS Profile

PMS appears as a complex tangle of symptoms caused by an imbalance in female hormones, primarily an excess of estrogen in relation to progesterone. Approximately three to ten days before menstruation, levels of progesterone fall, along with blood levels of calcium and magnesium. Progesterone, calcium, and magnesium all have relaxing effects on both the mind and body. When they are in short supply, symptoms such as irritability, muscle cramps, and insomnia occur. At the same time, levels of series-2 prostaglandins increase. These hormone-like substances provoke inflammation and muscle contractions and contribute to headaches, cramps, and joint pain. Blood-sugar levels drop, resulting in fatigue, food cravings, and poor concentration, and even immune function takes a nose-dive, making a woman more susceptible to colds, flus, and herpes outbreaks. All of these physiological shifts wreak havoc with the body and mind and cause the varied symptoms of PMS.

PMS SYMPTOMS

Abdominal bloating	Hot flashes
Acne	Indigestion
Backache	Insomnia
Breast tenderness	Irritability
Constipation	Joint pain
Depression	Mood swings
Fatigue	Muscle cramps
Food cravings	Nausea
Headache	Poor concentration
Heart palpitations	Water retention

Joanie is typical of women who suffer from PMS. When she was in her early thirties, she noticed that she felt irritable during the week before her menstrual period and found that she was easily annoyed with her family and work colleagues. She gained five pounds of water weight each month, craved chocolate insatiably, suffered from headaches, and was exhausted. Only when her menstrual flow started did her symptoms abate.

As happens for many women, Joanie's symptoms intensified as she entered her forties. Hormonal shifts in the premenopausal years often exacerbate PMS, and Joanie was miserable. She was desperate for relief, and adopted a healthier diet, cut out caffeine, began exercising daily, and took time for relaxation every day. To help to balance her hormones naturally, Joanie drank herbal teas made from *vitex* and *dandelion root,* made calming *chamomile* tea for tension relief, and drank *dandelion leaf* tea several days before menstruation to prevent fluid retention. For long-term energy building, she took *Siberian ginseng.* The first month, Joanie felt calmer and did not gain her usual five pounds of water weight. After three months, she felt only the slightest drop in energy around the time of her menstrual period; her other symptoms had virtually disappeared.

It wasn't very long ago that PMS was dismissed as purely emotional, and women who complained of symptoms were told that there was no physical basis for their complaints. Although it seems clear now that PMS is hormonally driven, there is still much to learn about this complex disorder. In most cases, many factors must be taken into account to effectively treat PMS, including diet, lifestyle, and emotions. While relieving symptoms is important, it is essential to bring balance into your life. If you focus only on symptom relief and ignore the underlying imbalances, PMS tends to worsen over time.

Balancing Your Hormones Naturally

Your liver is a key player in maintaining a healthy balance of hormones, which is essential for relieving PMS. One of the main functions of your liver is to detoxify and neutralize all harmful substances that enter your bloodstream, such as pesticides, pollutants, toxic fats, and metabolic by-products. This important organ is also responsible for detoxifying estrogen and helps to keep excess estrogen from accumulating in your body. Your liver can perform this task well only when it is not overburdened with other toxins. You can keep your liver healthy by eating organic foods, drinking pure water, and avoiding exposure to all chemicals and pollutants. Herbs are also helpful for improving liver function. Mild bitter herbs such as *dandelion root* and *burdock root* stimulate the flow of bile, which naturally cleanses the liver. In Chinese medicine, a congested liver is related not only to menstrual problems but also to irritability and mood swings, the classic picture of PMS. *Bupleurum,* a

Chinese herb, is often prescribed for treating PMS because it relieves liver stagnation. Bupleurum is the primary ingredient in a Chinese herbal formula called *Hsiao Yao Wan,* which is available in Chinese pharmacies, many natural foods stores, and also by mail-order.

For hundreds of years, women throughout the world have relied on herbs for balancing hormones and healing their reproductive organs. *Vitex (Vitex agnus-castus)* is one of the best herbs for relieving PMS symptoms and has been used for centuries in Europe as a tonic herb for nourishing the reproductive system. Vitex enhances the function of the pituitary gland, which in turn stimulates the production of progesterone. In addition, it has sedative and antispasmodic properties and inhibits prolactin, another hormone that exacerbates PMS. Vitex works best as a long-term herbal tonic and should be taken for at least six months to obtain the full benefits. The berries have a mild, peppery flavor and can be taken as a tea, in capsules, or as an extract. To make a tea, pour one cup of boiling water over two teaspoons of crushed vitex berries. Cover, steep for 15 minutes, strain, and drink three to four cups daily. You can also take one-half teaspoon of liquid extract or two capsules three times a day.

The following *Hormone-Balancing Tea* combines herbs that improve liver function with vitex. For best results, drink three cups daily for at least six months.

Hormone-Balancing Tea

3 teaspoons dandelion root

2 teaspoons burdock root

3 teaspoons vitex berries

2 teaspoons licorice root

1 teaspoon ginger root

4 cups water

Place herbs and water in a covered pot. Bring to a boil over medium heat, lower the heat, simmer covered over low heat for 15 minutes. Remove from heat and steep an additional 20 minutes. Strain, and drink 3 to 4 cups daily.

Herbal Remedies for Specific PMS Symptoms

A number of other herbs are helpful for relieving the uncomfortable symptoms of PMS, including headaches, water retention, insomnia, and mood swings. These herbs can be used as needed for symptom relief.

Water Retention: Diuretic herbs such as *dandelion leaf, parsley,* and *nettle* are excellent for safely relieving water retention. Because these herbs are rich in minerals, they do not deplete the body of potassium as do pharmaceutical diuretics which can cause dangerous electrolyte imbalances. Make a tea by pouring one cup of boiling water over two teaspoons of dried herb, cover, and steep for ten minutes. Strain, and drink three cups a day as needed.

Mood Swings: Gentle, calming herbs that can take the edge off tension include *chamomile* and *linden.* These make delicious mild teas and can be enjoyed as often as desired. For more severe mood swings, try *St. John's wort,* a potent and safe natural antidepressant. It takes approximately three months for St. John's wort to take full effect. Take one-half teaspoon of liquid extract or two capsules three times a day. In clinical studies that have proven the effectiveness of St. John's wort in treating depression, standardized extracts of the herb were used. If you want to use a standardized extract, take 300 milligrams three times daily of a product containing 0.3 percent hypericin, which is considered to be the active ingredient. For anxiety relief, *kava* is extremely effective. It not only eases anxiety, but also acts as a mild mood elevator and takes effect almost immediately. Take one-half teaspoon of liquid extract or two capsules three times a day. For more information on depression and anxiety, see Chapters 13 and 14.

Fatigue: For long-term energy building, take *Siberian ginseng.* It takes several months to feel the full benefits of the herb, but it slowly and steadily builds energy reserves while helping your body more easily adapt to both emotional and physical stressors. Take one-half teaspoon of liquid extract or two capsules twice daily for at least three months. For more information on fatigue, see Chapter 12.

Insomnia: For a mild case of occasional sleeplessness, try a cup of *passionflower* tea one hour before bedtime. Pour one cup of boiling water over two teaspoons of dried herb, cover, and let steep for ten minutes. For a more potent herbal sedative, try either *valerian* or *hops* extract. Take one-half teaspoon of either extract one hour before bed, and repeat the dosage if necessary. For more information on insomnia, see Chapter 15.

Headache: Ginger has anti-inflammatory properties and is often helpful for relieving headaches. To make ginger tea, simmer one to two teaspoons of fresh-grated ginger root in one cup of water in a covered pot for ten minutes. Strain, sweeten if desired, and drink three to four cups a day as needed. If you suffer from frequent headaches, see Chapter 19 for more detailed information.

Nutritional Help for PMS

While herbal remedies help to rebalance hormones and improve liver function, you'll obtain positive results more quickly if you also make a few simple changes in your diet and lifestyle. Certain foods upset hormonal balance, overburden the liver, and contribute to mood swings and fatigue. The primary offenders are refined carbohydrates and concentrated sugars, caffeine, alcohol, and polyunsaturated fats.

Eliminating all sources of caffeine is a good place to begin if you suffer from PMS. Caffeine stresses your liver, pancreas, and nervous system—as little as one cup of coffee a day is enough to cause PMS problems. I've known several women who discovered that simply giving up coffee was sufficient to banish their PMS symptoms. Caffeine is found not only in coffee, but also in black tea, chocolate, and certain over-the-counter medications including some sold to relieve PMS! The short-term burst of energy that caffeine provides is not worth the long-term detrimental effects. If you are looking for a natural energy boost, try Siberian ginseng, ginger, or green teas. Although green tea contains small amounts of caffeine, it has powerful health-enhancing properties and is generally well tolerated by most people. However, if you are especially sensitive to caffeine you should avoid green tea and drink Siberian ginseng tea or ginger tea instead.

Many women also crave sugar and chocolate during the week prior to menstruation because of the energy-boosting, calming, and slightly euphoric effects they provide. While giving in to the craving may provide temporary satisfaction, both sugar and chocolate upset blood-sugar levels and worsen PMS symptoms. Strong cravings for chocolate often indicate a need for more magnesium, and you may be able to assuage your chocolate cravings with healthier magnesium-rich snacks such as almonds and other nuts and seeds. Cravings for sweets often arise because of unstable blood-sugar levels and your body's need for an immediate source of energy. However, eating concentrated sweets exacerbates blood-sugar swings, and causes fatigue and mood disorders. Complex carbohydrates such as whole grains, legumes, potatoes, and fresh fruits are healthful sources of natural sugars that won't upset blood-sugar balance. The high-fiber content of complex carbohydrates also speeds the elimination of excess estrogen that has been broken down by the liver and prevents it from being reabsorbed into the bloodstream.

Proteins and healthful fats also help to maintain stable blood-sugar levels. Make sure to eat two servings of good-quality lean proteins such as fish, poultry, or tofu daily. If you eat meat or poultry, buy only that which is free of hormones. Most conventionally raised animals are treated with hormones, which adds to the load of excess estrogen in your body. For the same reason, be cautious when buying dairy products, and buy only those that are certified organic.

Foods rich in essential fatty acids such as cold-water fish (salmon, sardines, and mackerel), fresh raw nuts and seeds, freshly ground flaxseeds and flaxseed oil, avocados, and extra-virgin olive oil supply the building blocks for series-1 prostaglandins, the beneficial prostaglandins that help to balance hormones. Avoid all hydrogenated oils, such as margarine and vegetable shortening, and polyunsaturated supermarket oils such as safflower oil, corn oil, and sunflower oil. These unhealthy fats stimulate the production of problem-causing series-2 prostaglandins and also overburden the liver, which hinders detoxification.

You can help your liver in its task of neutralizing estrogen by adding plenty of antioxidant-rich foods to your diet. Dark leafy greens and deep yellow-orange vegetables and fruits are loaded with beta-carotene; citrus fruits, red peppers, and broccoli are high in vitamin C; whole grains and garlic are rich in selenium; and seafood and pumpkin seeds are good sources of zinc. Along with eating a diet abundant in antioxidant foods, taking a high-potency multivitamin and mineral supplement is a good idea to ensure consistently adequate levels of these health-protecting nutrients.

Supplements for Easing PMS

Vitamin B-6, magnesium, vitamin E, and gamma linolenic acid are among the most helpful supplements for balancing hormones and relieving PMS symptoms. Vitamin B-6, along with other B-complex vitamins, supports the liver in its job of breaking down and neutralizing estrogen. Research has shown that it helps to relieve premenstrual bloating and mood swings. Take 100 milligrams of B-6 daily in a balanced B-complex supplement.

Vitamin E, in the form of d-alpha tocopherol (400 to 800 units daily), helps to balance the ratio of estrogen to progesterone and can relieve PMS symptoms within a couple of months. While vitamin E is nontoxic, it does have a mild anti-clotting effect. If you have hypertension or a bleeding disorder consult with your health-care practitioner before taking large doses of vitamin E supplements.

If you have insatiable cravings for chocolate premenstrually, you may be deficient in magnesium. Chocolate is rich in magnesium, but the high fat, sugar, and caffeine content intensify PMS symptoms. Magnesium is needed by the liver to metabolize estrogen, and it also helps to stabilize blood-sugar levels. In addition, low levels of magnesium contribute to fluid retention. Try taking 400 to 800 units of magnesium daily along with 800 to 1,200 units of calcium. If you suffer from PMS-related insomnia, take at least half of your calcium-magnesium supplement about an hour before bed. Magnesium and calcium help to relax both the mind and body and promote restful sleep.

Gamma linolenic acid (GLA), an essential fatty acid that the body makes from linoleic acid, is also often helpful for relieving many PMS-related symptoms. GLA promotes series-1 prostaglandins and helps to normalize hormone production. Because a variety of factors (including aging) can interfere with the body's conversion of linoleic acid to gamma linolenic acid, many women are deficient in this essential nutrient. Supplements of GLA are available as evening primrose oil, black currant oil, and borage oil. Take enough capsules to equal 240 milligrams of gamma linolenic acid daily.

Other Natural Remedies for PMS

Regular exercise is essential for relieving both the emotional and physical discomforts of PMS. Exercise stimulates the production of endorphins, the body's natural mood elevating chemicals, and is one of the best therapies for depression, anxiety, and mood swings. Plan for at least 30 minutes of aerobic exercise four times a week. This is the minimum amount that will make a difference in the way you feel. Gradually increase the amount of time you spend exercising until you are engaged in some type of aerobic activity 45 minutes six times a week. Choose activities that appeal to you, such as brisk walking, hiking, biking, swimming, dancing, or skating, and vary what you do to avoid boredom. Yoga is also immensely helpful for relieving physical stress and calming the mind. Because emotional tension makes PMS much worse, the time that you dedicate to preventing and relieving stress will repay you many times over. Devote at least 15 minutes daily to meditation, deep-breathing exercises, and other forms of deep relaxation to decrease the production of stress hormones that cause physical imbalances. See Appendix II for a variety of relaxation, breathing, and meditation exercises. Allow yourself plenty of indulgences, too, in the form of aromatherapy baths, massages, and other ways of acknowledging that you deserve to treat yourself with love and respect.

The emotional aspects of PMS can be every bit as uncomfortable as the physical manifestions, if not more so. Talking with friends can serve as a release for pent-up emotions and provide reassurance that you are not alone in what you are feeling and that your symptoms are not "all in your head." It can be an immense relief just to acknowledge what you are feeling. Journaling can also be helpful in providing an avenue for exploring and releasing feelings. And, of course, good therapy can help tremendously if you suspect that there are emotional wounds that are contributing to your PMS symptoms.

Aromatherapy Treatments for PMS

Fragrant essential oils have a healing effect on the body and the mind and can be used in a variety of self-nurturing treatments for

relieving PMS. Clary sage, lavender, and rose geranium are all especially helpful for the complex emotional and physical symptoms that
characterize PMS.

Clary sage has a tranquilizing effect and is excellent for relieving nervous tension. While it is deeply relaxing, it also has an uplifting effect on the psyche. It helps to relax tense muscles and is
considered to be a hormone balancer. It has a sweet, musty fragrance and blends well with lavender.

Lavender has gentle soothing and relaxing effects and eases
tension, irritability, and fatigue. It relieves PMS-related headaches
and insomnia and also helps to regulate menstruation. Lavender has
a sweet, herbaceous floral scent and can be used alone or in combination with clary sage or rose geranium.

Rose geranium harmonizes both the mind and the body. It
helps to balance hormones and has antidepressant properties. Rose
geranium has an herbal rose fragrance with overtones of citrus and
blends well with lavender.

PMS-Relief Massage Oil

2 ounces almond oil

8 drops clary sage essential oil

16 drops lavender essential oil

1/2 teaspoon vitamin E oil

*Mix oils together, shake well, and store in a tightly capped dark-
glass bottle in a cool, dark place.*

Use this PMS-relief massage oil as often as you desire. You can
use it in massage treatments or apply a small amount after bathing
as an all-over body moisturizer. You can also use essential oils in
baths to ease PMS discomfort. Add four drops of clary sage or rose
geranium and eight drops of lavender essential oils to a bathtub of
comfortably warm water. Soak for 20 minutes, allowing yourself
time to deeply relax and to enjoy the benefits of the essential oils
on your body and your mind.

Natural Progesterone Therapy

While diet and lifestyle changes and herbal treatments are usually sufficient to relieve mild to moderate cases of PMS, more severe cases may benefit from natural progesterone therapy. It's best to consult with your health-care practitioner for guidance in using any type of hormone therapy.

Natural progesterone is different from synthetic progesterone in that there are no side effects associated with its use. Synthetic progesterone is well known for causing headaches, weight gain, and other unpleasant symptoms. Natural progesterone is available as both a cream that is applied to the skin and in tablet form. The cream is sold over the counter in some pharmacies and natural foods stores. Many women are confused about creams containing wild-yam extract that claim to be natural sources of progesterone. Wild-yam cream without added progesterone does not contain the active hormone. Progesterone is synthesized from wild yam, but it must undergo a laboratory process for conversion to progesterone. A progesterone cream must contain progesterone in order to be effective, and it will say so on the label.

When using a natural progesterone cream, apply approximately one-quarter teaspoon daily to areas where the skin is thinnest—on the abdomen, breasts, inner arms, and upper chest, rotating the areas of application daily. Most women use the cream continuously from one or two days before ovulation until the first day of menstruation, but some use it every day. Again, it's best to consult your health-care practitioner for guidance. While some women respond in the first month to natural progesterone therapy, for others it takes several months to gain the full benefits.

Chapter 4

Be Cramp-Free

More than half of all women experience dysmenorrhea, more commonly known as menstrual cramps. While for some women the cramping that accompanies menstruation is relatively mild and subsides after the first day of bleeding, other women suffer severe cramping that interferes with normal life for several days each month. Menstrual cramps not only cause abdominal discomfort, but can affect the whole body. Common symptoms include low-back pain, nausea, diarrhea, headaches, fatigue, abdominal bloating, vomiting, and dizziness.

Healing Menstrual Pain

Doctors classify menstrual cramps as either primary or secondary dysmenorrhea. While secondary dysmenorrhea is caused by a physiological problem such as endometriosis, uterine fibroids, or pelvic infection, there is no organic disorder associated with primary dysmenorrhea. But this doesn't mean that the pain you are feeling is imaginary. Until fairly recently, menstrual cramps were thought to be purely emotionally based. However, studies in the late 1970s showed that women who suffer from menstrual cramps have high levels of series-2 prostaglandins, hormone-like substances that trigger muscle contractions.

Series-2 prostaglandins cause uterine-muscle spasms that restrict blood flow to the pelvic area, which allows waste products such as lactic acid to accumulate. In Chinese medicine, menstrual cramps are regarded as a symptom of blood stagnation. The increase in estrogen levels that commonly occurs for women who are approaching menopause also contributes to menstrual cramping, especially dull, aching abdominal pain. High estrogen levels cause fluid retention, abdominal bloating and low-back pain.

If you suffer from sudden, severe cramping, consult your health-care practitioner to rule out a pelvic infection.

Nutrients That Reduce Pain-Causing Hormones

In most cases, menstrual cramps can be prevented with a healthful diet, regular exercise, and time out for relaxation. Herbs can help to regulate hormones and relieve cramps if they do occur, and massage and baths with essential oils relax the body and mind and help to ease the physical and emotional tension that contributes to cramping.

What you eat has a direct effect on your body's production of prostaglandins. While series-2 prostaglandins are a primary cause of menstrual cramps, series-1 prostaglandins have the opposite effect and help to relax the uterus. These hormone-like substances are made from fatty acids in the fats and oils you consume. Your body makes prostaglandins from both linolenic acid (omega-3 fatty acids) and linoleic acid (omega-6 fatty acids). Omega-3 fatty acids are found in fresh walnuts; cold-water fish such as salmon, sardines, and mackerel; and flaxseed and flax oil. Omega-6 fatty acids are found in vegetable oils, grains, seeds, and meats. Most women eat plenty of omega-6 fatty acids, but don't get enough of the omega-3 fatty acids. An excess of omega-6 fats in relation to omega-3 fats creates an imbalance that favors the production of series-2 prostaglandins. In addition, unhealthful fats such as hydrogenated oils, refined supermarket oils, and foods containing these oils such as crackers, chips, and baked goods stimulate the production of problem-causing prostaglandins.

To increase beneficial prostaglandins, be sure to eat foods rich in omega-3 fatty acids at least several times a week. If you suffer from intense menstrual cramps, you may want to supplement your diet with one tablespoon of cold-pressed flaxseed oil or two tablespoons of freshly ground flaxseeds daily. Taking supplements of gamma linolenic acid (GLA), an essential fatty acid that the body makes from linoleic acid, can also be helpful. Evening primrose oil, black currant oil, and borage oil are all good sources of GLA. Take enough capsules to equal 240 milligrams of GLA daily.

The dip in blood-calcium levels that occurs just before menstruation is another contributing factor to menstrual cramping. Calcium has a natural relaxing effect on the body, as does magnesium. Eat foods that are naturally rich in calcium and magnesium, such as dark leafy greens, seeds, nuts, beans, and legumes, and take a calcium-magnesium supplement that contains at least 1,000 milligrams of calcium and 400 milligrams of magnesium daily. Vitamin B-6 and vitamin E also have a positive effect on menstrual cramps. Vitamin B-6 has been shown to help the body produce the anticramping series-1 prostaglandins. Take 100 milligrams of B-6 daily in a balanced high-potency B-complex supplement and 400 units of natural vitamin E in the form of d-alpha tocopherol.

Banish Cramps with Exercise

Regular exercise helps not only to prevent cramps, but can also help to relieve them. Aerobic exercise stimulates circulation and encourages the production of endorphins, your body's natural pain-relieving chemicals. Try to schedule at least 30 to 45 minutes of aerobic activity such as brisk walking, biking, or dancing five or six days a week. Be sure to drink plenty of fluids, because dehydration can increase cramping. In addition to aerobic exercise, stretching exercises such as yoga gently increase circulation to the pelvic area and help to relieve the stagnation that contributes to cramping. While relaxing yoga poses can help to ease menstrual cramps, avoid upside-down poses such as the shoulder stand while you are menstruating. Yoga also facilitates deep relaxation, which brings the mind and body into balance. Creating a regular time for relaxation in the form of yoga, meditation, or deep-breathing exercises is helpful for relieving menstrual cramps, because emotional tension depletes your body of calcium and increases levels of series-2 prostaglandins. See Appendix 2 for suggestions for relaxation exercises.

Herbs for Relieving Menstrual Cramps

Herbs especially useful for treating menstrual cramps include anti-spasmodics such as *cramp bark* and *ginger,* sedatives such as *chamomile, valerian,* and *hops,* and anti-inflammatories such as *white willow.*

Cramp bark *(Viburnum opulus)* contains natural chemicals that help to relax tense uterine muscles. Used by Native Americans, cramp bark is one of the best herbs for relieving menstrual cramps. Although it is a powerful herb, it is safe to use over a long period of time. It can be made into a tea, but you may prefer taking it as a liquid extract or in capsules because it has a strong, bitter flavor. Take one-half to one teaspoon of extract or two capsules three to four times daily as needed. For severe cramps, take every two hours as needed until cramps subside.

Valerian *(Valeriana officinalis)* has been used for centuries as a safe, nonaddictive herbal sedative. It also has antispasmodic properties that help to relieve cramps. Valerian is especially helpful when cramps are accompanied by emotional tension or insomnia. Because of the intense earthy, pungent scent and flavor, most people prefer to use valerian root as a liquid extract or in capsules rather than as a tea. Take one-half to one teaspoon of extract or two capsules three to four times a day as needed. Note that while the majority of women find valerian deeply relaxing, about 5 percent react to the herb as a stimulant rather than as a sedative. If you find this to be true, try hops as an alternative.

Ginger *(Zingiber officinalis)* is excellent for stimulating circulation and relieves stagnation in the uterus by gently promoting menstrual flow. It also has antispasmodic properties that help to relax the uterine muscle. Fresh ginger root acts as a natural cramp preventative because it contains compounds that block the formation of trouble-making prostaglandins. Fresh ginger can be found in most supermarkets and makes a delicious, spicy tea. Simmer one to two teaspoons of fresh ginger root in one cup of water in a covered pot for five minutes. Remove from heat and steep covered for 10 minutes. Strain, sweeten if desired, and drink as often as needed. Ginger can also be used externally as a hot compress over the abdomen to stimulate circulation (see Appendix II), and in the form of essential oil in massage treatments. Ginger is a terrific remedy for relieving the nausea that sometimes accompanies menstrual cramps—try chewing on a piece of candied ginger or taking up to 10 capsules of dried powdered ginger as needed.

Chamomile *(Matricaria recutita)* is a gentle sedative and antispasmodic that relaxes the uterus and has mild tranquilizing effects. It makes a good-tasting tea and is helpful for mild cramps, especially when combined with ginger. Pour one cup of boiling water over two teaspoons of dried herb. Cover, steep for 10 minutes, strain, and drink as often as desired.

Hops *(Humulus lupulus)* has sedative properties similar to valerian and is also a muscle relaxant. It is a good choice for those who do not do tolerate valerian well and is excellent for promoting deep sleep. Because hops has a bitter flavor, most women prefer taking it as a liquid extract or in capsules. Take one-half to one teaspoon of extract or two capsules three times a day as needed.

White Willow *(Salix alba)* is sometimes called "herbal aspirin." In fact, the active ingredient in aspirin (salicylate) was originally derived from willow bark. Willow has mild anti-inflammatory and pain-relieving properties and has been used for centuries to relieve pain. Willow has a bitter, astringent flavor. To make a tea, simmer two teaspoons of willow bark in one cup of water in a covered pot for 10 minutes. Strain and drink up to three cups a day. As an alternative, take one-half to one teaspoon of liquid extract or two capsules three times a day as needed.

Gentle Cramp-Ease Tea

3 teaspoons fresh ginger root, grated
3 teaspoons chamomile
2 cups water

Simmer ginger root and water in a covered pot for 10 minutes.
Remove from heat and add chamomile. Cover and steep for 10
minutes. Strain, sweeten if desired, and drink as needed. For
more severe cramps, use the following Cramp Relief Formula.

Cramp Relief Formula

1 ounce cramp bark extract
1/2 ounce valerian or hops extract
1/2 ounce white willow bark extract
1/4 ounce ginger root extract

Combine extracts in a dark-glass bottle and shake well. Take 1/2
teaspoon of extract in a small amount of warm water every two
to three hours as needed to relieve menstrual cramps.

Prevent Cramps with an Ancient Chinese Herb

One of the best-known herbs from ancient China is dong quai
(Angelica sinensis), a root with an earthy, sweet flavor that is considered to be the most important tonic herb for women in the Chinese herbal pharmacy. Both Chinese and Western herbalists
prescribe dong quai to ease menstrual difficulties and maintain
reproductive health. Because dong quai has muscle-relaxing and
pain-relieving properties, it is helpful for easing menstrual cramps,
and it has an overall balancing effect on the reproductive system.
Researchers have identified phytoestrogens (plant hormones) in
dong quai that help to regulate hormones.

This popular herb is found in many herbal formulas for women. For best results, it should be taken over a long period of time—at least three to six months. Dong quai is nontoxic, but do not take it during menstruation, because it stimulates bleeding. Take the herb during the first two weeks of the menstrual cycle, discontinue the week before menstruation begins and during the week of menstruation, and then resume taking the herb when menstruation ceases. Dong quai is most commonly available as a liquid extract and in capsules. Take one-half teaspoon of extract or one capsule three times a day.

Aromatherapy Treatments for Easing Cramps

Herbs are excellent for relieving mild to moderate menstrual cramps, but more severe cramps call for extra help. Hot compresses placed over the abdomen, massage with essential oils, and hot aromatherapy baths relax tense muscles and bring circulation to the pelvic area. Several essential oils are especially helpful for easing cramps.

Marjoram has sedative and pain-relieving properties and also stimulates menstrual flow. It increases local circulation and relaxes the nervous system and the muscles. Marjoram has a warm, herbaceous, slightly sweet scent.

Lavender relieves nervous tension and is soothing and balancing. It also helps to regulate menstruation and has mild pain-relieving properties. Lavender has a floral, herbaceous, sweet fragrance.

Ginger has warming, stimulating properties that encourage sluggish menstrual flow. It is also an antispasmodic and helps to ease cramping. Ginger has a warm, spicy scent.

Massage approximately one teaspoon of the following oil over your abdomen and lower back twice a day to relieve cramps. You can intensify the action of the essential oils by placing a hot-water bottle over your abdomen. Hot compresses made from the same essential oil blend are also helpful. Add three drops of marjoram, four drops of lavender, and three drops of ginger essential oils to a basin of hot water. Soak a thin cotton dish towel in the water and wring it out. Place the hot, wet towel over your abdomen and cover with a thick, dry towel to retain the heat. Change the hot towel as soon as it begins to cool, replacing it with a fresh hot towel. Continue placing hot compresses over your abdomen for 15 to 30 minutes.

Cramp-Ease Massage Oil

2 ounces almond oil
6 drops marjoram essential oil
8 drops lavender essential oil
6 drops ginger essential oil
1/2 teaspoon vitamin E oil

Combine oils in a dark-glass bottle and shake well. Store tightly capped in a cool, dark place.

Hot baths are wonderful for relaxing the body and mind and easing cramps. Add ten drops of lavender and four drops of marjoram essential oils to a bathtub of comfortably hot water and soak for 20 minutes. For additional muscle-relaxing properties, add two cups of Epsom salts, which are rich in magnesium, a natural muscle-relaxing mineral. Hot sitz baths are also excellent for relieving uterine cramps (see Appendix II for directions). Add five drops of lavender essential oil and two drops of marjoram essential oil to the sitz bath if desired.

The Importance of Self-Nurturing

Oftentimes, menstrual cramps are a signal from your body that you need to slow down, go inward, and take time for self-nurturing. A healthful diet and regular exercise help to promote the production of beneficial prostaglandins and curtail the production of pain-causing prostaglandins, and herbs can help to both prevent and relieve pain. But it's still important to take a "time out" each month during menstruation. Menstrual cramps are an indication that something is out of balance in your hormonal and reproductive systems. Try paring down your daily responsibilities as much as possible and schedule time for a massage, a hot aromatherapy bath, or a quiet relaxing evening. Slowing down and taking time for self-nurturing gives your body the opportunity to come into balance and often yields remarkable results.

Sarah was 42 years old and had suffered from intense menstrual cramps from the time she began menstruating until she was in her late twenties. The cramps subsided after the birth of her first child, and she thought that she was finished with problematic menstrual cycles. She was dismayed in her early forties to find that the cramps had returned with a vengeance. Her cramping was so severe that she spent one day in bed each month, and she suffered from nausea, low-back pain, and headaches in addition to intensely painful cramps. As a mother of two teenagers and with a full-time law practice, Sarah was resentful of the intrusion that menstrual cramps made in her life. I suggested that she make dietary changes to help to balance her hormones and to start exercising several times a week, which she did. Sarah began taking dong quai and used the *Cramp Relief Formula* as needed. I encouraged her to take time out during her menstrual cycle for relaxation and to plan ahead for nurturing treatments. Sarah just wanted the pain to go away and had difficulty accepting that she needed to allow herself some "down time." She did notice some relief after three months of dietary changes, exercise, and herbs, but it was only when she began allowing time for self-nurturing that she experienced the most change. She scheduled a massage each month, took long, hot baths with essential oils, and relaxed with her favorite movies and a hot-water bottle on her abdomen on the first day of her menstrual cycle. While she still experienced some cramping at times, she no longer felt nauseous or debilitated.

Chapter 5

Nip UTIs in the Bud

At some point in life, most women will experience a urinary tract infection, commonly referred to as a bladder infection or cystitis. Doctors usually prescribe antibiotics to treat the infection, but natural treatments are almost always preferable to drug therapy. Antibiotics wipe out all bacteria in the body, including the friendly flora in the intestinal and genitourinary tracts that protect us against disease. It's a well-known fact that antibiotic treatment for urinary-tract infections sets a woman up for a rebound vaginal yeast infection. The link between UTIs and yeast infections is so well established that many doctors prescribe antibiotics and an antifungal cream simultaneously. Instead of relying on antibiotics, a more healthful approach is to strengthen the bladder against invading bacteria and to learn to recognize the symptoms of an impending infection so that you can take immediate action with herbal and other natural remedies.

Recognizing a Urinary Tract Infection

Feeling the need to urinate frequently and urgently, painful or burning urination, and pelvic pain are common symptoms of a bladder infection. You may also have a fever or blood in your urine. These symptoms, especially if accompanied by chills, nausea, and pain in the mid-low back may signal a more dangerous kidney infection. With any type of urinary tract infection, it's important to see your health-care practitioner for a bacterial culture and an accurate diagnosis. Kidney infections *must* be treated with antibiotics to prevent possible permanent and life-threatening kidney damage. A simple bladder infection can usually be successfully treated with herbs and other natural remedies, but you should schedule a return visit with your health practitioner for a follow-up bacterial culture about 10 days after starting treatment to make certain that the bacteria have been eradicated. Because an infection can continue without symptoms and cause serious damage, it's better to err on the side of safety.

With these cautions in mind, know that most urinary tract infections can be treated without antibiotics. Learning to recognize the early warning signs of a bladder infection and taking immediate action will enable you to take a natural approach to nipping urinary tract infections in the bud.

How to Support Your Body's Natural Defenses

Most urinary tract infections are caused by the bacterium *E. coli,* a normal inhabitant of the intestinal tract. These bacteria are eliminated from the body in bowel movements and are found around the anus. It's a short trip from the anus to the urethra, the urinary opening through which urine is passed from the body. If these bacteria migrate up the urethra and into the bladder, they can cause an infection.

Your body has several defensive strategies against bacterial invasion. Urine has a natural pH level that discourages bacterial growth, and normal urination washes away bacteria that try to ascend through the urethra. The interior of the bladder itself has natural antimicrobial properties, and if bacteria do begin to multiply, your immune system begins cranking out increased numbers of infection-fighting white blood cells. You can support your body's natural defenses by drinking plenty of fluids to increase urine flow and by using herbs and other natural remedies that bolster immune response and prevent bacteria from adhering to the lining of the bladder.

A Folk Remedy that Really Works

An old folk remedy that has been proven scientifically to prevent and relieve urinary tract infections is cranberry juice. For a long time, cranberry juice was thought to work by making the urine more acidic, which helps to discourage bacterial growth. But researchers now believe that cranberry juice relieves bladder infections because it makes the walls of the bladder slippery and prevents bacteria from gaining a foothold. For an infection to develop, bacteria must be able to adhere to the mucous membranes that line the bladder. Cranberry juice is especially helpful for preventing bladder infections, and if you are prone to UTIs, you might consider making cranberry juice a daily habit. It takes about 16 ounces of cranberry juice daily to protect the bladder from infection. Avoid supermarket brand juices, which are sweetened with large amounts of refined sugars. Sugar suppresses the immune system and also feeds the bacteria that cause infection. Buy unsweetened cranberry juice instead and dilute it with an equal amount of unsweetened apple juice. As an alternative, you can take supplements of cranberry extract, one capsule three times a day.

Other juices that are helpful for healing urinary tract infections are cucumber, parsley, and celery. All three are cooling and purifying for the urinary tract and their mild diuretic action increases urine flow and washes bacteria from the bladder. Drinking plenty of fluids is essential for both preventing and treating urinary tract infections. Strive for eight glasses of liquids daily, with half of that being pure water. If you feel the stirrings of an infection, you should double that amount. Choose from pure water, herbal teas, and unsweetened juices diluted with an equal amount of water. Avoid caffeinated beverages and alcohol because they irritate the urinary tract, and stay away from all sweetened beverages because they feed bacterial growth. For the same reason, you should avoid all concentrated sweeteners and refined carbohydrates when battling a urinary tract infection.

Eating one or two cups of yogurt daily that contains the beneficial *Lactobacillus acidophilus* organism will encourage a healthy population of the beneficial bacteria that help to keep problem-causing bacteria under control. You can also take supplements of probiotics, which are combinations of various beneficial flora in a concentrated form. Buy supplements that contain at least one billion viable *Lactobacillus acidophilus* and *Bactobacillus bifidum* bacteria per dose and take one or two capsules before breakfast for one month. If you do have to take antibiotics, be sure to take beneficial flora supplements to repopulate the healthy bacteria that are destroyed by the drug.

Other supplements that are especially helpful for treating a urinary tract infection include vitamin C, bioflavonoids, vitamin A, and zinc, all of which boost immune response and promote tissue healing. Take 4,000 milligrams of vitamin C combined with bioflavonoids in divided doses throughout the day during an active infection, and 25,000 units of vitamin A and 30 milligrams of zinc daily for up to two weeks.

Herbal Relief for UTIs

Herbs are excellent for treating urinary tract infections. I've found that herbs almost always prevent a full-blown infection, especially if they are used as soon as you notice the first symptoms of an infection. My first bladder infection caught me by surprise in my early twenties. I awoke in the middle of the night with an urgent need to urinate and was frightened by the intense burning and pain and the blood in my urine. I took antibiotics to fight the infection because I wasn't aware of herbal alternatives, but since that time I've successfully prevented several bladder infections by using herbs and natural remedies and have been able to avoid taking antibiotics.

Most of the herbs used for UTIs have diuretic properties, which means that they increase urine flow. This helps to flush the bladder of harmful microorganisms. Many of these herbs also have antimicrobial properties and help to directly combat the infection.

The following herbs are powerful and safe treatments for urinary tract infections.

Uva ursi *(Arctostaphylos uva ursi),* sometimes called bearberry, has been used by cultures as diverse as the Native Americans and the Chinese for treating urinary tract infections. Uva ursi contains a natural compound called arbutin, which is transformed in the urinary tract into hydroquinone, a potent urinary antiseptic that is effective against the *E. coli* organism. Uva ursi also has diuretic action and helps to cleanse the urinary tract. The antibacterial component of uva ursi seems to be most effective in an alkaline environment, so it may be helpful while using the herb to avoid cranberry juice, citrus, tomatoes, and other foods that might acidify the urine. Uva ursi has an astringent but not unpleasant flavor. Make a tea by pouring one cup of boiling water over two teaspoons of dried leaves. Steep for ten minutes, strain, and drink three cups a day. As an alternative, take one-half teaspoon of liquid extract or two capsules three times a day. Although uva ursi is safe when used in recommended amounts, don't exceed the recommended dosage or use it for more than two weeks, because in high doses it can cause nausea and irritate the kidneys. Do not take uva ursi during pregnancy.

Goldenseal *(Hydrastis canadensis)* is also a potent antimicrobial that contains a natural antibiotic called berberine that is effective against many strains of harmful microorganisms, including *E. coli.* In addition, goldenseal has anti-inflammatory and astringent properties that help to soothe inflamed mucous membranes. As with uva ursi, the natural antibiotic in goldenseal is most effective in an alkaline environment, so avoid eating acidifying foods while you are taking the herb. Pour one cup of boiling water over one teaspoon of powdered herb. Steep 10 minutes, strain, and drink three cups a day. Goldenseal is extremely bitter and is easiest to take as a liquid extract or in capsules. Take one-half to one teaspoon of extract or two to three capsules three times a day. Because it is a uterine stimulant, goldenseal should not be used during pregnancy.

Juniper *(Juniperus communis)* berries contain an aromatic oil that has antimicrobial and diuretic properties. It steps up the fluid-filtering rate of the kidneys, which increases urine output. Juniper has a sweet, pungent, and astringent flavor. To make a tea, pour one cup of boiling water over one teaspoon of crushed berries, cover, and steep for 20 minutes. Strain, and drink up to three cups a day. Overuse of juniper can irritate the kidneys, and the herb should not be used for more than four to six weeks at a time. If you have kidney disease or are pregnant, do not use juniper.

Marshmallow *(Althaea officinalis)* is a gentle diuretic that has mild immune-enhancing properties. While it won't fight infection as do uva ursi or goldenseal, it makes a soothing tea that helps to cleanse the bladder. Marshmallow has a pleasant, sweet flavor. Simmer one teaspoon of chopped dried root in one cup of boiling water in a covered pot for five minutes. Remove from heat and steep an additional ten minutes. Strain, and drink three to four cups throughout the day.

Other herbs that can be used to gently increase urine flow include *nettle, dandelion leaf,* and *parsley.* Make a tea by pouring one cup of boiling water over two teaspoons of dried herb (or two tablespoons of chopped fresh herb). Steep for 10 to 15 minutes, strain, and drink three to four cups daily.

The following formulas are most helpful when used at the initial stages of a bladder infection. For best results, use both the *Bladder Cleansing Tea* and the *Infection-Fighting Formula.* Continue taking both for several days after the symptoms abate to be sure that all of the harmful microorganisms have been eradicated.

Bladder Cleansing Tea

3 teaspoons marshmallow root
2 teaspoons dandelion leaf
2 teaspoons crushed juniper berries
3 teaspoons nettle
4 cups water

Simmer marshmallow root in water in a covered pot for 5 minutes. Remove from heat and add dandelion leaf, juniper berries, and nettle. Cover, and steep for 15 minutes. Strain, and drink 3–4 cups throughout the day.

Infection-Fighting Formula

1 ounce uva ursi extract
1/2 ounce goldenseal extract
1/2 ounce echinacea root extract

Combine extracts in a dark glass bottle and shake well. Take 1 teaspoon four times a day in a small amount of warm water.

Ease UTIs with Aromatherapy

Aromatherapy essential oils can be added to baths, compresses, and massage oils to help to relieve urinary tract infections. Sitz baths can ease the pelvic pain that sometimes accompanies an infection. See the directions for sitz baths in Appendix II, and add five drops each of juniper and sandalwood essential oils to the tub.

Juniper is a potent detoxifying oil with diuretic properties and is specifically an antiseptic for the urinary tract. It has a pungent, sweet, woodsy fragrance. Do not use juniper during pregnancy.

Sandalwood is also an antiseptic and diuretic and is used extensively in Ayurvedic medicine for treating urinary tract infections. It has a complex, rich, woodsy and sweet scent.

Tea tree is a potent antiseptic that directly kills the bacteria that cause urinary tract infections. If you suffer frequently from UTIs, add two drops of tea tree oil to one cup of warm water and use regularly as a genital wash after bowel movements and following intercourse. Tea tree oil has a pungent, camphor-like scent.

Aromatherapy Bath for UTIs

2 cups Epsom salts
1 cup baking soda
6 drops sandalwood essential oil
4 drops juniper essential oil

Fill bathtub with comfortably hot water, adding Epsom salts and baking soda while the tub is filling. Add sandalwood and juniper essential oils just before entering the tub. Soak for 15 to 20 minutes.

> ### Massage Oil for UTIs
>
> *1 ounce almond oil*
> *7 drops sandalwood essential oil*
> *5 drops juniper essential oil*
> *1/4 teaspoon vitamin E oil*
>
> *Combine oils and store in a dark glass bottle. Use as a massage oil over the abdomen and lower back.*

How to Prevent UTIs

A few simple precautions can help you avoid urinary tract infections. Good hygiene is essential for preventing UTIs. Always wipe from front to back to keep bacteria away from the urethra. Don't use scented toilet paper, perfumed or deodorant soaps, bubble bath, or feminine-hygiene sprays, all of which dry out the delicate vaginal tissues and make you more prone to infection. Wash thoroughly soon after sexual activity, and if you are prone to frequent urinary tract infections, rinse with a solution of one cup of warm water with two drops of tea tree oil to kill bacteria.

Drink plenty of fluids, especially pure water and herbal teas. Your need for fluids varies according to your diet, your level of activity, and the climate and season, but a good general guideline is to drink enough so that you need to urinate every couple of hours. This keeps your bladder cleansed and free of trouble-causing microorganisms.

Treating Chronic Interstitial Cystitis

My friend Tina thought she was suffering from recurrent bladder infections, but no infectious microorganisms could be found in her urinary tract. She was diagnosed with chronic interstitial cystitis, an irritation of the bladder that is not caused by infection. The symptoms are similar to a urinary tract infection and include an urgent need to urinate, frequent and painful urination, getting up at night to urinate, and pelvic pain that subsides after urinating.

No one knows for sure what causes chronic interstitial cystitis, but it's thought to be an autoimmune disorder, and food allergies may play a role. If you've been diagnosed with this problem, follow the general guidelines for preventing bladder infections. It's especially important to avoid substances that irritate the bladder, such as alcohol and all sources of caffeine. Stress-management therapies such as deep relaxation and visualization are helpful for calming the nervous system and stimulating the body's natural healing response. See the suggestions in Appendix II for relaxation and visualization exercises.

Chapter 6

Relieve Vaginal Infections Naturally

Almost every woman has battled a vaginal infection at one time or another, and some women seem to have a series of infections that never completely clear up. The changing hormones characteristic of the premenopausal and menopausal years make the vagina more susceptible to the opportunistic microorganisms that cause vaginal infections.

Most of the organisms that cause vaginal infections live in the vagina without causing problems. It's only when the healthy flora that inhabit the vagina are depleted or the normal slightly acidic vaginal pH balance is disrupted that the trouble-making organisms begin to grow out of control. A healthy immune system is essential for preventing opportunistic infections, and natural treatments based on herbs and essential oils help to fight off infectious microorganisms and restore a healthy balance to the internal environment.

Symptoms of Common Infections

It's important to learn to distinguish between the symptoms of a vaginal infection and healthy vaginal secretions. The vagina normally produces secretions that cleanse the mucous membranes, maintain a mildly acidic environment, and help to prevent infection. The color and consistency of this discharge varies throughout the menstrual cycle. Following menstruation, when hormone levels are low, there is very little vaginal discharge. As hormone levels increase, the vaginal discharge becomes creamy and is white or yellow in color. At ovulation, the discharge is clear, gel-like, and stringy, and may be tinged with blood. Following ovulation, the discharge again becomes white or yellow until menstruation.

Most vaginal infections are characterized by burning and itching of the vagina and vulva and an increase in vaginal discharge that may be an unusual color or odor. There may also be redness and swelling of the genitals. The discharge varies according to the type of microorganism causing the problem and provides clues as to the cause of the infection. *Always consult your health-care practitioner for a definitive diagnosis of the microorganism that is causing an infection.* Although many women feel comfortable self-diagnosing a simple yeast infection, it's a good idea to consult your health-care practitioner to rule out uncommon but serious vaginal infections such as chlamydia and gonorrhea. Attempts at self-treating these diseases can result in sterility and even death. In addition, always consult your doctor immediately in the case of symptoms accompanied by pelvic pain or fever, which are signs of possible pelvic inflammatory disease.

With these cautions observed, in the vast majority of cases there are three common organisms that cause most vaginal infections, and all can be treated with natural remedies.

Candida albicans is a normal inhabitant of the intestinal tract and vagina. It becomes troublesome only when an imbalance allows the organism to overpopulate the vagina. Symptoms include itching, redness, and a white, cottage cheese-like discharge that may have a yeasty odor. This is the most common type of vaginal infection, and almost every woman will have at least one yeast infection at some time in life.

There are both internal and external factors that make a woman susceptible to candida overgrowth. A candida infection is often caused by antibiotic use, which kills off the friendly flora in the body that normally keep the candida organism under control. Increased blood sugar levels caused by a high-sugar diet, diabetes, pregnancy, and higher estrogen levels in the premenopausal years also make a woman more susceptible to candida infections. Many women find that they are prone to yeast infections around menstruation, because hormonal fluctuations and menstruation change the vaginal pH. Following menopause, yeast infections are more likely because of lower hormone levels and a decrease in the production of protective vaginal mucus. External factors that contribute to candida infections include tight clothing and synthetic underwear, deodorant soaps and feminine hygiene products, and chlorinated hot tubs and swimming pools.

Bacterial vaginosis is the second most common vaginal infection and is a generic diagnosis for infections caused by organisms other than candida albicans or trichomonads. Because bacterial vaginosis is usually caused by the bacteria *Gardnerella vaginalis,* it is often referred to as gardnerella. Like candida, gardnerella is another case of the overgrowth of an organism commonly found in the vagina. Symptoms include a gray or yellowish discharge with a foul or fishy odor. There may also be itching, irritation, lower-back pain, and painful urination. Bacterial vaginosis often recurs in women who have been treated with antibiotics. The key is not to try to eradicate the organism, but instead to focus on strengthening the immune system and improving the health of the vagina so that the organism cannot cause problems.

Trichomonas vaginalis is caused by a single-celled protozoan called trichomonad. This is also a common vaginal infection and will affect about one out of every five women. Symptoms include a yellow or greenish frothy discharge that may be blood-tinged, with a foul or fishy odor. The genitals tend to be swollen and inflamed, with burning and itching. If the organism infects the bladder, it can cause frequent, burning urination. However, some women have no symptoms at all and discover that they have the infection only during a routine gynecological exam. Trichomonas is thought to be transmitted sexually, but it can take years to develop after exposure. It is more difficult to treat than a yeast infection, but will generally respond to a concentrated treatment program that includes infection-fighting and immune-building herbs.

Herbal Healing for Vaginal Infections

Herbs applied externally ease the inflammation and itching of vaginal infections. Internally, herbs bolster the body's immune response and directly fight the microorganisms that are causing the infection. Use both external and internal treatments for best results, and be patient. It may take a couple of weeks for full recovery from a vaginal infection. When you use herbs and other natural remedies for treating a vaginal infection, you are not only fighting the infection, but you are also strengthening your body against future infections. Prescription and over-the-counter drugs that are used to treat vaginal infections treat only the symptoms and do nothing to help restore a healthy balance to your vagina or to strengthen your immune system.

Paula, one of my students, fought recurrent yeast infections for years. Her doctor suggested that she use an over-the-counter medication as needed, but Paula was tired of battling constant infections. She began using *echinacea* and *garlic* to strengthen her immune system, drastically cut back on her sugar intake, and took baths in *thyme, calendula,* and *lavender* to soothe her inflamed and irritated vaginal tissues. It's been two years since she's had a yeast infection, and she continues to eat raw garlic regularly and to monitor her sugar intake to keep her body in balance.

The following herbs are among the most helpful remedies for treating vaginal infections.

Echinacea *(Echinacea purpurea)* helps to fight infection by bolstering your body's natural immune response. Take one-half teaspoon of extract or two capsules four to six times a day until the infection subsides.

Garlic *(Allium sativum)* is a powerful antimicrobial that directly fights bacteria, fungi, and other microorganisms that cause infection. Garlic must be eaten raw and either chopped or chewed to take full advantage of its infection-fighting properties. However, chewing a raw clove of garlic is not easy for most people because it is so pungent. Try finely chopping a garlic clove and adding it to salad dressings, pasta, or soups just before serving, or simply wrap the chopped garlic in a small piece of bread to make it easier to take. For general immune enhancement, eat one clove daily. During an active infection, eat three cloves daily.

Goldenseal *(Hydrastis canadensis)* has natural antibiotic properties and has been proven to kill a wide variety of harmful microorganisms. In addition, goldenseal has astringent properties that soothe inflamed mucous membranes. Goldenseal can be used both internally and externally. To fight an infection, take one-half to one teaspoon of liquid extract or two to three capsules of goldenseal three times a day. Do not use goldenseal during pregnancy, because it may stimulate uterine contractions. Goldenseal can also be used as a vaginal wash (see following instructions).

Thyme *(Thymus vulgaris)* is rich in fragrant essential oils that have potent antimicrobial properties. When made into a strong tea and applied externally, it relieves itching and is excellent for baths and vaginal washes for treating vaginal infections. Pour four cups of boiling water over six tablespoons of thyme, cover, and steep until cool. Strain and use in a sitz bath or as a vaginal wash (see following instructions).

Calendula *(Calendula officinalis)* is a soothing, gentle herb that calms inflammation and promotes tissue healing. It also has antimicrobial properties (including antifungal action) and is ideal for vaginal washes. Pour four cups boiling water over six tablespoons calendula, cover, and steep until cool. Strain and use as a vaginal wash.

Herbal Vaginal Wash

2 tablespoons powdered goldenseal

3 tablespoons thyme

3 tablespoons calendula

4 cups boiling water

Pour boiling water over herbs, cover, and steep until cool. Strain through a coffee filter. Use as a vaginal wash several times a day, or as a gentle douche twice daily.

Some health practitioners caution against douching because of the possibility of forcing microorganisms up into the uterus, which can potentially cause pelvic inflammatory disease. Too frequent douching can also alter the pH balance of the vagina, making it more susceptible to the overgrowth of harmful microorganisms. It's probably safer to soak in a warm sitz bath, allowing the water to flow into the vagina naturally. If you choose to douche, do so very gently.

Aromatherapy Treatments for Vaginal Infections

Many essential oils have infection-fighting properties and are helpful for treating vaginal infections. They can easily be added to baths, sitz baths, and vaginal rinses to help ease uncomfortable symptoms such as itching, inflammation, and discharge. In general, use approximately ten drops of essential oil in a sitz bath and five drops to one quart of warm water for a vaginal rinse or douche.

Lavender has soothing and healing properties and relieves itching and inflammation. Although gentle, it is a potent antimicrobial. It has a sweet, floral, herbaceous fragrance.

Tea tree has powerful antiseptic properties and kills a wide variety of infectious microorganisms. Always dilute tea tree oil before using it on tender mucous membranes such as the vagina. Tea tree oil has a pungent medicinal scent reminiscent of eucalyptus.

Relieve Symptoms with Herbal Sitz Baths

Warm or hot herbal sitz baths help to relieve itching, pain, and inflammation and also help to wash out the vagina. Make a strong herbal tea to add to the bath by pouring one quart of boiling water over four tablespoons each of calendula and thyme. Steep until cool, and strain. Pour the tea into a large plastic tub (large enough to hold your buttocks) and fill with enough hot water so that the water barely reaches your navel when you are sitting in the tub. Your upper body and your legs will be out of the tub. The idea is to soak just your pelvic region in the water. Add 10 drops of lavender essential oil. Soak for 15 minutes, allowing the water to flow freely into your vagina. Repeat this bath twice daily until the infection has subsided.

Restore Healthy pH with Apple-Cider Vinegar

Apple-cider vinegar is an excellent way to relieve itching and helps to restore a healthy pH balance to the vagina. Mix three tablespoons of unpasteurized apple-cider vinegar with one quart of warm water. Add three drops of lavender essential oil and two drops of tea tree essential oil. Use as a vaginal rinse as needed, or as a gentle douche twice daily.

To soothe irritated mucous membranes, apply a liberal amount of aloe vera gel or calendula gel or salve to the vaginal tissues two or three times daily. For directions for making homemade calendula salve, see page 11.

Prevent Infections with a Low-Sugar Diet

The most important dietary change you can make to help prevent and relieve vaginal infections is to cut down on your intake of sugar and other sweeteners. Sugar not only suppresses immune function, but it also directly feeds the microorganisms that cause infection, especially the candida organism. A diet high in sugar and refined carbohydrates disrupts the healthy acidity of the vagina and sets the stage for infection.

For most women, it's not realistic nor is it necessary to eliminate sweets entirely. But, in general, make an effort to limit the number of sweets you eat and choose the best quality. As much as possible, satisfy your sweet cravings with fresh fruits, which offer health-protective benefits along with their sweet taste. However, if you have an active vaginal infection, avoid all sources of concentrated sweeteners, including fruit juices, honey, and maple syrup until the infection is completely eradicated.

To help to replenish the healthy bacteria that keep unfriendly microorganisms under control, eat yogurt that contains live acidophilus cultures every day. Studies show that eating one cup of yogurt daily reduces the incidence of vaginal infections by more than half. If you have taken antibiotics, or if you are prone to recurrent vaginal infections, take a supplement that provides live *Lactobacillus acidophilus* organisms. Buy capsules that contain at least one billion viable organisms each, and take two capsules before breakfast for two months. If you have an infection, you can also help to restore the population of healthy vaginal flora by inserting one or two capsules of powdered acidophilus into the vagina every night for two weeks. The capsules will dissolve overnight, releasing the beneficial flora into the vagina.

General Guidelines for Avoiding Infections

Vaginal infections are opportunistic infections and take hold when your immune system is weak or your internal environment is out of balance. The key to preventing vaginal infections is to strengthen your immune function and to restore a healthy balance to your vaginal environment in the ways outlined earlier. You can also help to prevent vaginal infections by practicing good hygiene and avoiding harsh chemicals such as those found in deodorant soaps, personal-hygiene sprays, scented toilet paper, and deodorant tampons and menstrual pads. These chemicals dry out delicate vaginal tissues and disrupt the balance of healthful bacteria. Avoid tight-fitting clothing and synthetic underwear, which promote the breeding of unhealthful microorganisms, and wash your underwear in hot, soapy water. If you have had an infection, wash your underwear in chlorine bleach to kill microorganisms and to prevent reinfection.

Chapter 7

Eliminate Fibroid Problems

Uterine fibroids affect up to half of all women and are one of the primary reasons for hysterectomies. In the majority of cases, though, natural treatments can help a woman avoid such drastic measures. Fibroids are a benign overgrowth of muscle tissue within the uterus or within the uterine wall. The presence of any type of abnormal growth can be frightening, but it is important to know that fibroids are not cancerous, nor are they associated with a higher incidence of uterine cancer. Common symptoms of fibroids include heavy bleeding during menstruation, irregular menstrual periods, and sometimes pelvic pain. While these symptoms may be uncomfortable, they are generally not harmful. More serious symptoms include anemia caused by heavy menstrual blood loss and bowel or bladder discomfort if the fibroids grow in such a way that they put pressure on the intestines or bladder. If there is not an immediate health threat, you have time to experiment with dietary changes, herbs, and other natural remedies to shrink the growths. Consult with your health-care practitioner, preferably someone who takes a holistic approach to your well-being and is willing to take the time to consult with you about alternative approaches to surgery.

Taking a Natural Approach to Fibroids

Because fibroids are stimulated by estrogen, if they become problematic they typically do so in the perimenopausal years when fluctuating hormones spur their growth. Multiple fibroid growths are common, and while they may be as tiny as the head of a pin, they can grow to the size of a grapefruit, or even larger. Many women have no symptoms at all and discover that they have fibroids only during a routine gynecological examination. Fibroids generally do not present a health crisis, and even though some doctors will try to rush a woman into a hysterectomy, there are good reasons for taking a "wait-and-see" approach. It's not uncommon for women who choose dietary changes, herbs, and other natural therapies to find their fibroids shrinking.

Eileen was diagnosed with fibroids in her late twenties, but they caused her no significant problems. However, when she was almost 40, increasing levels of estrogen typical of the pre-menopausal years spurred her fibroids to grow, and she began having pain, heavy menstrual bleeding, and some abdominal discomfort. Eileen adamantly did not want surgery and was highly motivated to make changes in her life that would help her body come back into balance so that the fibroids would shrink naturally. She changed her diet to reduce the excess estrogen in her body, took *vitex* to help balance her hormones, *dandelion* and *milk thistle* to improve her liver function, applied compresses several times a week to stimulate circulation to her uterus, and practiced a visualization technique where she imagined the fibroid tumors shrinking and dissolving. After several months, Eileen's doctor told her that the fibroids were shrinking, and while she still has the tumors, she has no noticeable symptoms.

Although it's unlikely that natural therapies will completely dissolve fibroids, they can many times help a woman avoid surgery. A compelling reason for avoiding surgery is that once a woman reaches menopause, fibroids almost always disappear naturally as estrogen levels decline. If you have fibroids and they are not causing you undue difficulties, experimenting with a natural approach to shrinking them and relieving symptoms is appropriate. However, be sure to check with your health-care practitioner for an evaluation at least once a year. If you experience an increase in bleeding, pain, or uncomfortable pressure in your abdomen, consult your doctor.

Regulate Hormones with Diet and Exercise

Because fibroids are stimulated by high-estrogen levels, adjusting your diet to decrease estrogen levels is essential. Avoid all foods that increase estrogen, such as saturated fats, hydrogenated fats, refined carbohydrates, and meat and dairy foods, especially those that have been commercially raised and given hormones.

Center your diet around vegetables, whole grains, legumes, fruits, nuts and seeds, and lean proteins such as fish and poultry that have been raised without hormones. If you eat dairy products, use only small amounts, and buy organically produced products to ensure that they are free of hormone residues. Avoid all foods treated with chemical pesticides and herbicides because they have dangerous hormonal effects on body tissues. Whenever possible, buy organically grown foods and drink filtered water. Include soy products such as tofu, tempeh, and miso in your daily diet; these are rich in plant hormones and help to naturally regulate estrogen levels. See page 297 (Appendix: How to Cook for Health) for a variety of delicious ways to prepare soy foods. Make a conscious effort to increase the amount of fiber in your diet, which should be easy if you are eating plenty of whole grains, legumes, fresh vegetables, and fruits. A high-fiber diet helps your body eliminate excess harmful estrogen.

Dietary supplements that are useful for treating uterine fibroids include vitamin C and bioflavonoids, which help to strengthen capillaries and alleviate heavy menstrual bleeding. Take 3,000 milligrams of vitamin C with mixed bioflavonoids daily in divided doses, and emphasize foods that are rich sources of vitamin C, such as citrus fruits, dark-green leafy vegetables, and tomatoes. To help your liver metabolize estrogen more efficiently, take a high-potency B-complex vitamin daily. It takes approximately six months to see results from making dietary changes. Be patient and persistent and

know that the changes you make will benefit not only your reproductive health, but your overall health as well.

Aerobic exercise such as brisk walking, bicycling, and dancing
is also extremely beneficial for reducing excess estrogen levels. Regular exercise eases the emotional and physical tension that contribute to hormonal imbalances and improves overall circulation.
Plan for a minimum of 30 minutes four times a week, increasing as
you comfortably can to 45 minutes six times a week.

In addition to diet, exercise, and herbs, natural progesterone
therapy, as discussed on page 23, can help to balance excess estrogen levels by increasing levels of progesterone. If you are interested
in using natural progesterone, consult your health-care practitioner
for guidance.

Herbal Help for Uterine Fibroids

The basis of an herbal approach to treating uterine fibroids is to
help to balance hormone levels and to improve liver function,
which helps to detoxify excess estrogen. In addition, herbs can help
to relieve symptoms caused by fibroids such as excessive bleeding
and cramping.

Vitex *(Vitex agnus-castus)* helps to normalize estrogen levels
by stimulating the production of progesterone. For the greatest benefit, vitex should be taken for at least six months. To make a tea,
pour three cups of boiling water over two tablespoons of crushed
vitex berries. Steep for 20 minutes, strain, and drink three cups a
day. Vitex has a spicy, peppery taste. You can also take one-half
teaspoon of liquid extract or two capsules three times daily.

Dandelion root *(Taraxacum officinale)* stimulates bile flow,
which helps to gently decongest the liver and improves liver function. It also has mild laxative properties, which encourages the elimination of excess estrogen. For best results, take dandelion for at
least three months. To make a tea, simmer three tablespoons of dandelion root in three and one-half cups of water for 15 minutes in a
covered pot. Remove from heat and let stand for an additional 15
minutes. Strain, and drink three cups a day. Dandelion root has an
earthy, slightly bitter flavor. You can also take one-half teaspoon of
liquid extract or two capsules three times daily.

Milk thistle *(Silybum marianum)* is a potent liver-protective herb that stimulates the growth of healthy new liver cells and improves the ability of the liver to detoxify estrogen. For best results, take an extract of milk thistle standardized for silymarin, which is considered to be the primary active ingredient. Take 140 milligrams of silymarin three times daily for at least three months. If you prefer to use the whole herb, you can grind milk thistle seeds in a coffee grinder and sprinkle them on cereals, salads, or other dishes. Eat approximately two tablespoons daily.

Nettle *(Urtica dioica)* is an excellent general health tonic. Rich in iron and other minerals, nettle builds healthy blood and is helpful for relieving anemia caused by excessive menstrual blood loss. Nettle is safe and gentle and can be taken indefinitely. To make a tea, pour three cups of boiling water over two tablespoons of dried nettle, cover, and steep for 15 minutes. Strain, and drink three cups daily. Nettle tea has a rich, pleasant flavor.

Yellow dock *(Rumex crispus)* is an excellent detoxifying herb. It improves liver function by stimulating bile flow and has mild laxative properties. Yellow dock is high in iron and helps to improve blood quality if anemia is a problem. To make a tea, simmer two tablespoons of dried root in three and one-half cups of water for 15 minutes in a covered pot. Remove from heat and allow to steep for an additional 10 minutes. Strain, sweeten if desired, and drink three cups daily. Yellow dock has a bitter, earthy flavor. If you prefer, you can take one-half teaspoon of liquid extract or two capsules three times a day.

Uterine Fibroid Tea

2 teaspoons dandelion root

2 teaspoons yellow dock root

2 teaspoons ginger root

2 teaspoons licorice root

3 teaspoons vitex berries, crushed

3 teaspoons nettle

4 cups water

(continued)

> *Simmer dandelion root, yellow dock root, ginger root, and licorice root in water in a covered pot for 15 minutes. Turn off heat, and add vitex berries and nettle. Cover, and steep for 20 minutes. Strain, and drink in equal portions 15 minutes before meals 3 times a day.*

If you prefer the convenience of taking herbs as an extract, you can use the same proportions for the tea to make a blend of extracts. Mix the extracts together in the proportions given and take one teaspoon in a small amount of warm water three times daily.

Herbs for Problematic Fibroids

Herbs can help to alleviate uncomfortable symptoms caused by uterine fibroids. However, before attempting self-treatment, have your doctor evaluate fibroids that cause pain or excessive bleeding.

Yarrow *(Achillea millefolium)* contains astringent compounds that constrict blood vessels and helps to curtail excessive blood flow during menstruation. For this purpose, yarrow should be taken several days before menstruation begins and throughout the menstrual cycle. To make a tea from yarrow, pour one cup of boiling water over one tablespoon of dried yarrow tops. Cover, and steep for 15 minutes. Strain, sweeten if desired, and drink three cups daily. Yarrow tastes astringent and slightly bitter. If you prefer, you can take one-half teaspoon of liquid extract or two capsules three times a day. Because yarrow has a stimulating effect on the uterus, it should not be used during pregnancy.

Cramp bark *(Viburnum opulus)* helps to relax muscle spasms, including uterine cramps. It also has astringent properties that help to reduce excessive blood loss. Simmer two teaspoons of the dried bark in one cup of water for ten minutes. Strain, and drink up to three cups a day. Cramp bark has a bitter, unpleasant taste. You may prefer taking one-half teaspoon of liquid extract or two capsules three times a day.

Aromatherapy Treatments for Fibroids

Essential oils increase circulation to the pelvic organs, relax tense uterine muscles, ease cramps, and encourage a state of overall relaxation that promotes healing. Use the following essential oils in sitz baths, massage oils, and abdominal compresses.

Ginger is a potent circulatory stimulant with warming properties. It also helps to improve liver function. Ginger has a spicy, warm scent.

Marjoram has potent sedative properties and is an excellent muscle relaxant that eases uterine cramps. It also has mild laxative action and helps to relieve constipation when used as an abdominal massage oil. Marjoram has a spicy, herbaceous, slightly sweet fragrance.

Rose is gentle and relaxing, and helps to ease physical and emotional tension. It has mild hormone-balancing properties and is considered to be a uterine tonic. Rose has a deep, sweet, floral fragrance.

Massage Oil for Fibroids

10 drops ginger essential oil
10 drops rose essential oil
2 ounces almond oil
1/2 teaspoon vitamin E oil

Pour oils into a dark-glass bottle. Store tightly capped in a cool, dark place, and shake well before using. Use as a massage oil over the abdomen and lower back.

Stimulate Healing with Sitz Baths

Sitz baths help to move blood into the pelvic area, which improves circulation and relieves the stagnation that contributes to the development of uterine fibroids. For best results, sitz baths should be used five times a week. Natural therapies take time and effort, but the results are well worth it.

Alternating hot and cold sitz baths are the most effective type of sitz bath for increasing energy flow to the uterus. The hot bath dilates the blood vessels and brings fresh blood to the pelvic region, while the cold water constricts the blood vessels and forces the blood out of the pelvis. The alternating dilation and constriction creates a surge of circulation that cleanses and nourishes the uterus. You'll need two plastic tubs that are large enough to sit in comfortably. Fill one tub with water as hot as you can tolerate, and the other with ice-cold water. You'll need to fill the tub only halfway or less with water—you'll be able to determine how much water you need by sitting in the tub. It usually takes a bit of experimentation to get the amount of water and the temperature just right. The hot tub should be approximately 105–110 degrees F, and the cold tub should be between 55 and 65 degrees F. You may need to add ice cubes to the cold tub to obtain the desired temperature. To increase the healing benefits of the bath, add five drops of ginger or marjoram essential oil to the tub of hot water.

Begin by lowering your buttocks into the hot tub—the water should feel uncomfortably hot at first. Sit with your upper body and your legs out of the tub, and make sure that your pelvic region is covered up to your navel with the water. Stay in the water for three minutes and then immediately move to the cold tub for one minute. Alternate between the hot and cold tubs three times, remaining in the hot tub each time for three minutes and the cold tub for one minute. Finish with the cold tub, towel off briskly, and rest for a few minutes, concentrating on the healing energy circulating in your pelvis.

How to Engage Your Imagination for Healing

Any time you deeply relax, you encourage the flow of healing energy throughout your body. Regularly practicing some form of deep relaxation encourages hormonal balance, strengthens your immune function, and eases the muscle tension that constricts circulation and energy flow. Take at least 15 minutes once or twice daily to practice deep relaxation (see suggestions in Appendix II for various relaxation exercises). Other ways of enhancing energy flow include yoga, tai chi, and massage. Experiment with these various practices to discover what feels good to you, and include one or more on a regular basis in your life.

You can consciously direct healing energy to your uterus by using visualization exercises. Use a form of deep relaxation that appeals to you, and when you are completely relaxed, imagine that with each inhalation, you are breathing pure, white light into your pelvis. Imagine the white light completely filling your pelvis, bathing and warming your reproductive organs. Focus on your uterus, and see the healing white light encircling and flowing into your uterus. Visualize your fibroid tumors dissolving as they are enveloped by the white light. Complete your visualization by imagining your uterus as pink, healthy, and normal. Practice this simple visualization exercise at least twice daily.

You may find as you practice deep relaxation or visualization that emotions rise to the surface of your conscious awareness. Don't ignore or suppress these feelings—they are coming to you for a reason and have a message for you. Acknowledge what you are feeling, and listen to your inner wisdom for clues to the ways that you may be suppressing your needs and desires. Abnormal growths such as fibroids can be a sign that there is some way that you are blocking your growth in the outside world. How might you be holding yourself back? What emotions are you not expressing that need to be expressed? What deep needs do you have that are not being met? These are not easy questions to answer, but be patient, give yourself the time for self-exploration, and use tools such as journaling, dream work, and therapy to help you to access your inner wisdom.

Chapter 8

Healing Cervical Dysplasia

Cervical dysplasia is the term used to describe abnormal cell growth on the cervix, the lower part and neck of the uterus that is the entrance to the uterus. Risk factors for cervical dysplasia include sexual activity at an early age (before age 18), multiple sexual partners, smoking, birth-control pills, and exposure to herpes simplex type II (genital herpes) and human papillomaviruses (venereal warts). In addition, a variety of nutritional deficiencies are clearly associated with an increased incidence of cervical dysplasia.

Don't Be Alarmed by Cervical Dysplasia

A diagnosis of cervical dysplasia is frightening for most women because of the association between cervical dysplasia and cervical cancer. The vast majority of women with cervical dysplasia do not develop cancer. However, cervical dysplasia should not be ignored, because if it is not treated it can progress and lead to cancer. The presence of cervical dysplasia is discovered through a Pap smear, a routine gynecological procedure that takes a sampling of cells from the surface of the cervix. These cells are examined under a microscope for abnormalities and are graded on a numerical scale from 1 to 4, with higher numbers indicating greater abnormalities. While the accuracy of Pap smears is controversial, it is still a helpful screening procedure, and stricter standards are making test results more reliable. If your test results come back positive for cervical dysplasia, you should request another Pap smear to rule out the possibility of error. You can also request a colposcopic exam, a painless procedure during which your physician examines your cervix with a lighted magnifying lens.

If you have stage-3 or -4 dysplasia, you should be treated by a physician. Standard treatments are effective and employ methods for removing the abnormal tissue, such as freezing, burning, laser, or surgery. In some cases, stage-3 cervical dysplasia can be treated with natural remedies, but this should be attempted only under the close supervision of your health-care practitioner. Although cervical dysplasia does not usually progress quickly to a cancerous state, it can.

Stage-2 cervical dysplasia is considered mild, and many doctors favor monitoring the condition while giving the body time to heal itself. In many cases, cervical dysplasia disappears on its own. But the appearance of abnormal cells is a clear message that you need to pay attention to your physical and emotional needs. On a physical level, you might need to clean up your diet, take time for relaxation and exercise, and strengthen your immune system. On an emotional level, you might find it helpful to take time for meditation, journaling, or other inner work that helps you understand this message from your body.

In any case of cervical dysplasia, it's important to rule out an underlying vaginal infection that may be causing the cell abnormalities. If there is an infection, clearing it up is often all that is needed to heal the dysplasia. If you choose to treat cervical dysplasia naturally, it is essential that you be monitored closely by your health-care practitioner. Follow the following program for one month and have another Pap smear. If the results are normal, you can discontinue the program, but you should still have a Pap smear every three months for one year. It may take up to three months to completely clear dysplasia, but you should be seeing positive results after one month.

Continue to have a Pap smear every month to monitor your progress while you are in the process of healing cervical dysplasia.

Taking a Natural Approach to Cervical Dysplasia

My friend Helen was diagnosed several years ago with cervical dysplasia. Her doctor wanted to perform laser surgery to remove the abnormal tissue, but Helen refused. She believed that the unhealthy cells in her cervix were related to a variety of emotional and physical stressors, and she wanted to have the opportunity to help her body heal naturally. Because her dysplasia was not severe, her physician agreed that she could postpone treatment. Ellen changed her diet, eliminating harmful foods and focusing on foods rich in cell-protecting nutrients. She added supplements such as antioxidants and folic acid, which are known to protect the cervix, and she began a daily program of walking and meditation to ease physical and emotional tension. In one month, her follow-up Pap smear showed that her cervical cells were healthier, but still showed signs of abnormal cells. Ellen began taking herbs to boost her immune function as well as using herbal treatments to heal her cervix. Her next Pap smear, one month later, was completely normal.

Powerful Nutrients That Reverse Abnormal Cell Growth

In any condition of abnormal cell growth, it is especially important to avoid those foods that are known to cause unhealthful cell changes, such as fried foods, polyunsaturated and hydrogenated oils, artificial additives and preservatives, and foods treated with hormones, pesticides, and herbicides. Center your diet around fresh vegetables, whole grains, lean proteins, and fresh fruits. Fresh vegetables and fruits are particularly helpful because of their high concentrations of antioxidant vitamins and minerals. Try to eat at least six servings of fresh vegetables and fruits every day, emphasizing dark leafy greens and deep-yellow-orange vegetables and fruits, which tend to be the richest sources of antioxidant compounds.

Deficiencies of a variety of nutrients are clearly associated with a higher incidence of cervical dysplasia and cervical cancer. Studies of women with cervical dysplasia show that they have low blood concentrations of antioxidants and folic acid and that supplementing with these nutrients can reverse the abnormal cell growth. If you have been diagnosed with cervical dysplasia, take 10 milligrams of folic acid daily for up to three months, along with a high-potency vitamin B-complex supplement. After a normal Pap smear or three months (whichever comes first) cut back to just the high-potency B-complex, and be sure to eat dark leafy greens daily, which are rich natural sources of folic acid.

High levels of antioxidants are also critical for protecting cells and preventing abnormal cell growth. As a general daily antioxidant supplement, take 25,000 units of beta-carotene with mixed carotenoids, 2,000 milligrams of vitamin C, 200 micrograms of selenium, and 400 units of vitamin E.

Herbs for Relieving Cervical Dysplasia

The most important herbs for treating cervical dysplasia are those with immune-enhancing and hormone-regulating properties. In addition, herbs that improve liver function help to naturally regulate hormones and promote detoxification, which is essential when working with any condition of abnormal cell growth.

Astragalus (*Astragalus membranaceus*) has been used for centuries in China as an immune-strengthening herb. It improves immune function in a number of ways, including stimulating the activity of white blood cells that gobble up abnormal cells. Astragalus has a mild, sweet, pleasant flavor and makes a tasty tea. Simmer 3 tablespoons of dried shredded astragalus root in three and one-half cups of water for 15 minutes in a covered pot. Remove from heat and let steep for an additional 15 minutes. Strain, and drink three to four cups daily. You can also take one-half teaspoon of astragalus liquid extract or two capsules three times daily. Astragalus can be taken indefinitely and is most effective for strengthening immune function when it is taken for three months or longer.

Vitex (*Vitex agnus-castus*) helps to gently normalize hormone levels. Vitex works best when it is taken for at least three months, and preferably six months. Vitex has a slightly peppery flavor. Make a tea by pouring one cup of water over two teaspoons of crushed berries. Cover, and steep for 15 minutes. Strain, and drink three to four cups daily. You can also take one-half teaspoonful of vitex extract or two capsules three times a day.

Burdock *(Arctium lappa)* is a gentle detoxifying herb that helps to bring the body into a state of balance. It improves digestion and liver function, has mild diuretic and laxative properties, and is rich in nutrients. Burdock has a rich, earthy flavor. To make a tea, simmer two tablespoons of burdock root in three and one-half cups of water in a covered pot for 15 minutes. Remove from heat and let steep for an additional 15 minutes. Strain, and drink three to four cups daily. If you prefer, take one-half teaspoonful of burdock extract or two capsules three times a day.

Dandelion *(Taraxacum officinale)* is one of the best liver-cleansing herbs. The bitter flavor gently stimulates bile flow, which naturally improves liver function and helps to purify the blood and bring hormones into balance. Dandelion root also has mild laxative and diuretic properties, both of which promote tissue cleansing. To make a tea, simmer two tablespoons of dandelion root in three and one-half cups of water in a covered pot for 15 minutes. Remove from heat and let steep for an additional 15 minutes. Strain, and drink three to four cups daily. You can also take one-half teaspoonful of extract or two capsules three times a day.

For greatest benefit, make a tea from a combination of these herbs to stimulate immune function, enhance detoxification, and bring hormones into balance.

Tea for Cervical Dysplasia

3 teaspoons astragalus root
3 teaspoons vitex berries
2 teaspoons dandelion root
2 teaspoons burdock root
2 teaspoons ginger root
4 cups water

(continued)

Place herbs and water in a covered pot and bring to a gentle simmer over low heat. Simmer 15 minutes, remove from heat, and allow to steep until cool. Strain, sweeten if desired, and drink 3 to 4 cups daily.

Herbal Treatments That Enhance Healing

Herbal treatments applied directly to the cervix can help to stimulate local immune function and heal damaged tissue.

Calendula *(Calendula officinalis)* has antimicrobial properties and helps to fight infection that may be contributing to cervical dysplasia. It also stimulates healing and has gentle astringent properties that soothe inflamed tissues. To make a tea to use as a douche, pour one quart of boiling water over 4 tablespoons of dried calendula blossoms. Cover, and let steep until cool. Strain before using.

Chaparral *(Larrea tridentata)* is a desert shrub with potent antioxidant and anticancer properties. It also has antiseptic action and is a natural herbal antibiotic. Chaparral leaves can be made into a tea for using as a douche, but they contain a lot of resin, which leaves a sticky residue on cooking pots and utensils. Using chaparral extract is easier. If you want to make a tea, simmer four tablespoons of chaparral leaves in one quart of water in a covered pot for 15 minutes. Remove from heat, cool to room temperature, and strain. If you are using the liquid extract, add one teaspoon to one quart of warm water.

Goldenseal *(Hydrastis canadensis)* is a powerful natural antimicrobial that is effective against a wide range of infectious microorganisms. It also has strong astringent action and helps to heal irritated tissues. To make a tea from goldenseal to use as a douche, pour one quart of boiling water over four teaspoons of powdered goldenseal. Cover, and steep until cool. Strain before using. Powdered goldenseal also makes an effective treatment when made into a pessary that is inserted into the vagina. Note that berberine, the ingredient in goldenseal responsible for its yellow color and for many of its healing properties, will stain anything it comes into contact with.

Vaginal Pessary for Cervical Dysplasia

1/2 cup cocoa butter
1/8 cup powdered goldenseal
1/8–1/4 cup powdered slippery elm bark
5 drops tea-tree essential oil
10 drops lavender essential oil

Melt cocoa butter in a small saucepan over low heat. Remove from heat and add goldenseal, stirring well. Add enough slippery elm bark to make a stiff paste. Add essential oils and mix thoroughly. Roll into small cylinders approximately the size of your little finger, place on waxed paper, and refrigerate until hardened. Store in a glass or plastic container in the refrigerator. To use, insert one pessary deep into the vagina every evening before bed. The pessary will gradually melt at body temperature. Use a menstrual pad to prevent staining clothing or bedding.

Herbal Douche for Cervical Dysplasia

4 tablespoons calendula flowers
1 teaspoon chaparral extract
5 drops lavender essential oil
1 quart water

Pour boiling water over calendula flowers, cover, and steep until lukewarm. Strain, and add chaparral extract and lavender essential oil. Use daily as a douche.

For best results, use the pessary at night, followed by the herbal douche in the morning. Repeat this treatment for five days in a row, rest for two days, and then repeat again for up to twelve weeks until the cervix has returned to normal.

Using Visualization to Access Healing Energy

A diagnosis of cervical dysplasia offers you an opportunity to go within to discover the deeper message that your body is giving to you. For many women, cervical dysplasia is a wake-up call that helps them to pay more attention to their needs. To get in touch with your inner wisdom, give yourself time for quiet reflection. Journaling, meditation, and time alone in nature can help you realize the truth about what you need for your healing to occur.

Visualization is a powerful tool for bringing your body into balance and accessing healing energy. Seeing your reproductive organs as perfectly healthy helps to bring your vision into reality. To help you create a clear image, look for pictures of a healthy uterus. You might also want to draw a picture of your uterus and cervix in a state of perfect health.

Set aside time to access your healing energy by taking a few minutes for a relaxing visualization two or three times a day. Close your eyes, take a slow, deep breath, and exhale completely. Imagine a warm, healing light circulating in your pelvis, bathing and cleansing your reproductive organs. In your imaginal journey, if you see any areas of unhealthy cells, visualize healing light soothing and purifying the tissues. Clearly visualize your uterus and cervix as pink and healthy. Spend a couple of minutes holding this image in your mind. Throughout the day, call upon this healing image and affirm to yourself that your cervix is completely healthy. See Appendix II for a more thorough discussion of visualization exercises.

Chapter 9

Ease Fibrocystic Breast Discomfort

Almost three-quarters of women have some degree of breast lumpiness, known in medical terminology as "fibrocystic breasts." Symptoms of fibrocystic breasts include swelling, tenderness, pain, and lumps that vary in size throughout the menstrual cycle, particularly during the week or two prior to menstruation. A woman's breasts are composed of milk glands, connective tissue that supports the glands, and fat. For most women, breast composition changes with age as the ratio of connective tissue to fat increases and the connective tissue becomes thicker and more fibrous. Until fairly recently, fibrocystic breasts were labeled as a disease, but because the condition is so prevalent it is now regarded as a normal variation in breast tissue.

Understanding Fibrocystic Breast Condition

Fibrocystic breast condition is broken down into three subtypes: fibrosis, cysts, and duct hyperplasia. Fibrosis is a thickening of the fibrous connective tissue that supports the milk glands. Fibrosis may be painful and may be accompanied by cysts. Cysts occur when tissue surrounding a milk duct overgrows, which blocks the duct and prevents it from draining normally. The milk duct swells, becoming a tender, fluid-filled sac that ranges in size from the head of a pin to a walnut or larger. Duct hyperplasia is an overgrowth of the lining of the milk duct, and is the only fibrocystic condition that is related to an increased risk of breast cancer. Finding a breast lump is a frightening experience, and it is important to have any breast lumps or changes in breast tissue evaluated by your health-care practitioner. As a note of reassurance, know that more than 90 percent of breast lumps are benign.

Although fibrocystic breasts are a common condition and cannot appropriately be labeled as a disease, they are a signal that most likely that there is an imbalance in your body chemistry. Breast pain, swelling, and lumpiness tend to worsen in the week or two prior to menstruation and appear to be caused by an excess of estrogen in relation to progesterone and also to an increase in prolactin, the hormone that prepares the breasts for potential pregnancy each month. Factors that influence estrogen and prolactin levels include a high-fat diet, caffeine, smoking, excess weight, and emotional stress. I have known many women who have completely reversed painful fibrocystic breast conditions through lifestyle changes and natural therapies.

Patti, a nurse practitioner in her early forties, suffered terribly from fibrocystic breasts for more than a decade. During the week preceding menstruation, her breasts were so painful that she wore a support bra even while sleeping and often resorted to strong pain-killing drugs. She was surprised to learn that she could heal her breast pain with natural therapies. Patti was willing to try a natural approach and even gave up caffeine (a prime contributing factor to fibrocystic breasts), which she relied on for a "jump start" in the morning and again in the afternoon when her energy began to flag. She also began taking supplements and herbs that specifically help to balance hormones. It took about four months, but Patti completely eliminated her breast pain and swelling and has not had any recurrences of cysts in the two years since she began making health-affirming changes in her life.

Dietary Guidelines for Balancing Hormones

The primary goal in relieving a fibrocystic breast condition is to reduce the levels of estrogen in the bloodstream that overstimulate hormone-sensitive breast tissue. You can take immediate action to lower your estrogen levels through adopting a dietary strategy that helps your body cut back on the production of estrogen and at the same time encourages the elimination of excess estrogen. Avoid saturated fats, polyunsaturated oils such as safflower, sunflower, and corn oil, and hydrogenated and partially hydrogenated oils. Use extra-virgin olive oil instead, a healthful monounsaturated fat that has been found to have a protective effect on breast tissue. Also include foods rich in omega-3 fatty acids, such as cold-water fish (salmon, sardines, mackerel) and flaxseeds or flaxseed oil. Center your diet around vegetables, fruits, whole grains, legumes, nuts, seeds, and lean proteins. Soy foods, such as tempeh, tofu, and miso and cruciferous vegetables, such as broccoli, cabbage, kale, and cauliflower, help to prevent estrogen from binding to and stimulating unhealthy growth in breast tissue. See Appendix: How to Cook for Health for a variety of recipes that feature these helpful foods.

Increasing fiber is essential for helping your body to successfully eliminate estrogen. Studies show that vegetarian women excrete two to three times more estrogen than women who eat meat, which is a good reason to increase the amount of vegetables, grains, and fruits in your diet. It is also critical to avoid all sources of dietary estrogen, such as meats and dairy products that have been commercially raised and subjected to hormones. Whenever possible, buy organically grown foods. Pesticides and herbicides are clearly linked to unhealthful hormonal changes in body tissues.

Caffeine is strongly associated with fibrocystic breast conditions; studies show that more than 90 percent of women with fibrocystic breasts improve when they forgo all sources of caffeine, which includes not only coffee, tea, and chocolate, but also decaffeinated coffee and tea (which still contain traces of caffeine), colas and other caffeinated soft drinks, foods with coffee flavoring such as candies and ice cream, and over-the-counter medications that contain caffeine.

Supplements that help to relieve fibrocystic breasts include vitamin E, which helps to normalize hormones, and vitamin B-complex, which helps the liver to detoxify excess estrogen. Take 400–800 units of vitamin E in the form of d-alpha tocopherol daily and a high-potency 50 to 100 milligram vitamin B-complex. Women with fibrocystic breast disease often respond favorably to supplements of gamma linolenic acid (GLA), an essential fatty acid that helps to regulate hormones. The body has to convert omega-6 fatty acids to gamma linolenic acid, and because a number of factors (including aging) interfere with this conversion, GLA is often in short supply. GLA supplements in the form of evening primrose oil, black currant seed oil, and borage seed oil are readily available. Take enough capsules to equal 240 milligrams of GLA daily. It usually takes at least three months to see results from taking GLA. After your breast tissue has returned to normal, cut the dosage in half and continue taking the supplement indefinitely.

How to Help Your Body Eliminate Toxic Estrogen

To help establish healthy flora in the intestinal tract, which improves bowel function and promotes the elimination of excess estrogen, take supplements of the beneficial flora *Lactobacillus acidophilus*. Buy supplements that provide one to two billion live organisms daily, and take one or two capsules before breakfast daily for one month. Eating yogurt that contains live *Lactobacillus acidophilus* organisms also helps to nurture beneficial flora in the intestinal tract. If constipation is a problem, take supplemental fiber in the form of powdered psyllium or pectin. Take one to three teaspoons of supplemental fiber in half a glass of liquid before breakfast or before going to bed at night. Follow with an additional glass of water. Fiber supplements can be taken indefinitely, but be sure to drink extra water when taking them to avoid creating constipation. You should be drinking plenty of pure water on a daily basis anyway to help your body eliminate toxins.

Drinking fluids such as water and herbal teas also helps your body to eliminate excess fluids that contribute to premenstrual breast swelling and tenderness. Drink at least six to eight glasses of water or herbal teas every day. Gentle cleansing herbal teas such as *dandelion leaf* or *nettle* have mild diuretic properties, and drinking up to three cups throughout the day can help to alleviate water retention. Make a tea by pouring three cups of boiling water over two tablespoons of dried herb. Cover, and steep for ten minutes. Strain, and drink throughout the day. Avoid excess salt, especially in the week or two prior to menstruation when water retention is most likely to occur. Foods such as asparagus, parsley, watercress, cucumber, cranberries, and watermelon also have diuretic properties and can help to relieve premenstrual water retention.

Herbal Relief for Fibrocystic Breasts

Poor liver function is strongly related to fibrocystic breast conditions because the liver is responsible for detoxifying estrogen. When the liver is not functioning up to par, excess estrogen accumulates in the bloodstream and causes unhealthful changes in hormone-sensitive breast tissue. Sluggish bowel function also allows excess estrogen that was on its way out of the body to be reabsorbed into the bloodstream. Herbs help to relieve fibrocystic breasts by improving liver and bowel function, as well as by helping to balance hormones through stimulating the production of progesterone.

Dandelion *(Taraxacum officinale),* both the root and the leaf, are helpful for treating fibrocystic breasts. The root stimulates bile flow and improves liver function, while the leaf is a powerful and safe diuretic that relieves the water retention that causes swollen, tender breasts.

Burdock root *(Arctium lappa)* is a traditional liver-cleansing herb that gently stimulates and enhances liver function.

Yellow dock root *(Rumex crispus)* contains potent bitter principles that act as a powerful liver cleanser. It also has laxative properties that help to cleanse the intestinal tract.

Vitex *(Vitex agnus-castus)* helps to regulate hormones by stimulating the production of progesterone, which brings estrogen levels into balance.

Prickly ash *(Zanthoxylum americanum)* stimulates circulation, including lymphatic circulation, helping to relieve the stagnation that contributes to the formation of cysts.

The following tea will enhance liver function, help to bring hormones into balance, improve lymphatic circulation, and relieve water retention. This formula has a bitter flavor, and you may prefer to take it as an extract. You can buy liquid concentrated herbal extracts and combine them in the same proportions given in the following recipe. Take one teaspoon of extract three times a day diluted in a small amount of warm water. It may take three months or even longer to improve a fibrocystic breast condition. After symptoms are relieved, cut back your dosage of either the tea or extract so that you are taking the formula only during the week prior to menstruation.

Herbal Tea for Fibrocystic Breasts

2 teaspoons dandelion root

2 teaspoons burdock root

1 teaspoon yellow dock root

3 teaspoons vitex berries

2 teaspoons prickly ash bark

2 teaspoons dandelion leaf

4 cups water

Simmer the dandelion root, burdock root, and yellow dock root in water in a covered pot for 15 minutes. Remove from heat, add vitex berries, prickly ash bark, and dandelion leaf, cover, and steep for an additional 20 minutes. Strain, sweeten if desired, and drink 3 to 4 cups daily.

Healing Breast Massage and Herbal Compresses

Hot and cold compresses and gentle breast massage improve circulation in breast tissue and are a wonderful way of caring for your breasts. Many women avoid touching their breasts because they are fearful of finding disease. Use your daily breast massage as an opportunity to affirm that your breasts are healthy. To ease pain, make compresses from anti-inflammatory herbs such as *chamomile, calendula,* and *yarrow.* Essential oils with anti-inflammatory properties such as lavender and chamomile are also helpful for easing breast pain, and essential oils such as grapefruit and lemon stimulate lymphatic flow. As a preventive measure, avoid wearing underwire bras because they restrict the normal healthy circulation of blood and lymphatic fluid.

Pain-Relieving Breast Compress

2 teaspoons chamomile flowers
2 teaspoons calendula flowers
2 teaspoons yarrow flowers
1 1/2 cups water
10 drops lavender essential oil
2 washcloths
hot water bottle

Pour boiling water over herbs, cover, and steep for 10 minutes. Strain, and add lavender essential oil. Dip washcloth into hot herbal solution, wring out slightly, and place over the breast. Cover with a dry towel and a hot water bottle to retain heat and leave in place for 3 minutes. Remove washcloth and replace with a second washcloth that has been dipped in cold water. Leave cold washcloth on breast for one minute, and immediately follow with the hot washcloth that has again been dipped into the hot herbal solution. Reheat the herbal solution if necessary. Repeat cycle 3 times, ending with the cold washcloth.

Healing Breast Massage Oil

2 ounces almond oil
1/2 teaspoon vitamin-E oil
15 drops lavender essential oil
5 drops grapefruit essential oil

Blend oils together in a tightly capped dark glass bottle. Apply approximately 1/2 teaspoon of oil to breasts immediately after bathing, while skin is still slightly damp. Massage breasts with a gentle, circular motion, finishing with sweeping movements, stroking from the breasts to the underarms to enhance lymphatic flow.

Chapter 10

Menopause: An Opportunity for Renewal

For most women, menopause is one of the most significant events that occurs at midlife. Many times, menopause coincides with other life challenges, such as children leaving home, transformations in career and relationships, and the aging or death of parents. This is a tremendous amount of change for a woman to adjust to, not only physically, but mentally, emotionally, and spiritually.

How well you adjust to these changes is greatly within your control. While hormonal fluctuations are an undeniable part of menopause, many of the unpleasant symptoms commonly associated with menopause are caused or exacerbated by poor eating habits, lack of exercise and rest, and emotional stress. A healthful diet, moderate exercise, plenty of rest, and reducing emotional stress all help your body adjust to hormonal changes with a minimum of discomfort. Herbs are wonderful allies during menopause: They help to regulate hormones, restore vitality, and provide relief from uncomfortable symptoms. Above all, self-nurturing is essential during menopause. The more attention you pay to your well-being, the better you will feel.

Understanding Your Changing Body

Most women begin experiencing the hormonal fluctuations that precede menopause by the time they reach their mid-forties, a time referred to as perimenopause. By the age of 55, the majority of women will have completed menopause. Common health concerns attributed to these hormonal shifts include hot flashes, weight gain, vaginal dryness, osteoporosis, depression, insomnia, fatigue, memory loss, and diminished sexual vitality. But many of these conditions are primarily caused by the accumulation of years of less than optimal living habits. It's important to realize that you can make changes at any time that will help you feel better, look better, and live longer.

COMMON MENOPAUSAL SYMPTOMS

Hot flashes
Vaginal dryness
Irregular heavy menstruation
Urinary tract infections
Heart palpitations
Sleep disturbances
Osteoporosis
Memory loss
Depression
Joint pain
Irritability
Anxiety
Loss of muscle tone
Weight gain
Dry skin
Cold hands and feet

Understanding what is happening in your body gives you the power to make informed choices as to how best to approach the changes you are experiencing. While menopause refers to the final menstrual period, it is more accurately a time of transition that encompasses the perimenopausal years through the year or two following the final menstrual cycle. Every month during your reproductive years, your ovaries produce estrogen and progesterone. Estrogen is made during the first half of your menstrual cycle to stimulate the growth of the uterine lining. At midcycle, the ovaries release a mature egg that travels down the fallopian tube into the uterus. During the two weeks following ovulation, the ovaries produce progesterone as well as estrogen, which prepares the uterus for possible pregnancy. If pregnancy does not occur, the ovaries stop making hormones, causing a sharp decrease in estrogen and progesterone levels. As a result, the uterine lining deteriorates and is shed during menstruation. By the time you are in your mid-forties, ovulation typically becomes erratic and hormones begin to fluctuate. Menstrual periods become irregular, sometimes occurring more frequently and sometimes less, with bleeding sometimes heavy and sometimes light. Most women find that their menstrual periods are initially more frequent and heavier and later become further apart and lighter in flow. It's also common to skip a month or two and then resume menstruating.

Not only do your ovaries produce estrogen and progesterone, but they also make other hormones called androgens such as testosterone and DHEA, which are important for maintaining muscle tone, sex drive, and overall well-being. After menopause, the ovaries no longer produce egg cells and they greatly decrease secretion of estrogen and progesterone. But they continue producing androgens, which take over the job of keeping you healthy. Androgens are also made by other organs and glands such as the adrenal glands. As the ovaries decrease their production of estrogen and progesterone, the amount of androgens made by other sources throughout the body increases. Another important role of androgens is that they are converted by fat cells in the hips and thighs to estrogen, which becomes an important source of this necessary hormone. This is a good reason to avoid being excessively thin, especially when entering the menopausal years.

The Key to Vitality

When your ovaries slow down their production of hormones, your adrenal glands step in to fill the gap. Although they don't generate anywhere near the amount that the ovaries once did, healthy adrenals do produce enough hormones to ease the transition through menopause and maintain lifelong vitality. The adrenals, small glands that sit just above the kidneys, play a primary role in physiological responses to physical and emotional stressors. However, our bodies were not meant to endure the chronic tension that many of us live with on a daily basis. As a result of trying to maintain balance under conditions of recurring stress, the adrenals become exhausted. Many factors deplete adrenal health, including environmental and physical stressors such as exposure to environmental toxins, physical or mental overwork, insufficient sleep, illness or injury, and even excessive exercise. Chronic emotional stress such as anxiety, depression, and fear also places a tremendous strain on the adrenal glands and is a primary cause of adrenal exhaustion.

Women who enter menopause with depleted adrenals have a more difficult time because their adrenals are not able to produce the small amounts of estrogen necessary for vitality. Common symptoms of adrenal depletion include fatigue, low blood sugar, insomnia, sugar cravings, depression, impaired memory, poor concentration, and frequent infections. Fortunately, the adrenal glands can be rejuvenated. To strengthen your adrenals, eliminate caffeine, sugar, and refined foods and make sure your diet includes plenty of lean proteins such as chicken, fish, turkey, and tofu. Eat frequent small meals to keep blood-sugar levels stable, and take a high-potency multivitamin and mineral daily. The B-complex vitamins, vitamin C, and herbs such as *Siberian ginseng* are especially helpful for adrenal health. Stop overworking, and allow yourself sufficient sleep and rest. Go to bed before 10 P.M. at night, because the sleep you get before midnight is the most restorative for the adrenals. Moderate exercise is helpful for reducing physical and emotional tension, but avoid overexercising and strive for a moderate approach that leaves you feeling energized, not exhausted, afterward. This may be easier said than done, but give yourself permission to slow down and to take time for self-nurturing. Carefully consider how you are spending your time and your energy, decide what obligations and commitments are really worthwhile or necessary, and eliminate the rest. In a nutshell, think of your adrenals as an energy bank, and concentrate on making fewer withdrawals and more deposits in the form of rest, relaxation, healthful foods, supplements, and herbs.

Taking a Natural Approach to Menopause

Conventional medicine relies on hormone-replacement therapy (HRT) for treating the uncomfortable symptoms of menopause as well as for preventing cardiovascular disease and osteoporosis in postmenopausal women. In general, the combination of estrogen and progesterone prescribed in HRT is effective for hot flashes, vaginal dryness and thinning, and depression, and it does appear to offer protection from cardiovascular disease and osteoporosis. However, many women do not feel good when taking synthetic hormones and report side effects that include breast soreness, bloating, nausea, acne, and headaches. HRT is also associated with an increased risk of dangerous blood clots, high blood pressure, gallbladder disease, and cancer, particularly breast cancer. For these reasons, many women prefer not to take synthetic hormones. There are natural hormones available now that have much less risk of unpleasant side effects, and hormone prescriptions can be tailored to an individual woman in the precise combination of estrogen, progesterone, and androgens that she needs. If you choose to explore hormone-replacement therapy, consult a naturopathic physician or other doctor who practices a holistic approach to health.

For the majority of women, the recommendations in this chapter will be sufficient to ease the transition through menopause without drugs and will help you to enter the second half of your life with health and vitality. A natural approach to menopause concentrates on improving overall health through diet, nutritional supplements, herbal tonics, exercise, rest, and relaxation, all of which help to bring the body into balance. For any uncomfortable symptoms that do arise, herbs, essential oils, and other natural remedies can help to ease your discomfort.

Dietary Guidelines for Menopause

What you eat influences how you feel on a daily basis and also lays the foundation for your health in the postmenopausal years. Researchers are finding that specific foods have a measurable effect on hormone levels, particularly foods that are rich in phytoestrogens. Phytoestrogens are plant compounds with mild estrogenic properties. Although phytoestrogens are estimated as being 50 times weaker than estrogen, they are helpful for balancing conditions of both estrogen excess or deficiency. Because they are similar to the hormones in your body, phytoestrogens bind to receptor sites in the body that estrogen normally occupies. If you are suffering from the effects of too much estrogen (which is the cause of many menopausal complaints such as hot flashes), phytoestrogens help to lower your blood levels of estrogen. If, on the other hand, you have too little estrogen (which contributes to osteoporosis), phytoestrogens provide some estrogenic activity and help to protect against bone loss.

Phytoestrogens are found in abundance in foods such as legumes, whole grains, nuts, flaxseeds, and apples. The phytoestrogens in soy are of special interest to researchers because Japanese women typically have a much easier transition through menopause than American women, and many experts believe that the Japanese reliance on soy as a dietary staple is the reason. Another benefit of plant estrogens is that while synthetic estrogen is related to an increased incidence of cancer, phytoestrogens appear to decrease the risk of reproductive cancers. Soy is easy to include in your daily diet in the form of tofu, tempeh, soy milk, miso, and tamari (a natural soy sauce). Add tofu or tempeh to sandwiches, salads, pasta dishes, and stir-fries, and use soy milk on cereal and in beverages. Miso and tamari are excellent for seasoning soups, stews, and sauces. See Appendix I for a variety of delicious ways to incorporate soy foods into your cooking repertoire.

Other helpful foods during the menopausal years include foods rich in omega-3 and omega-6 essential fatty acids, which help to keep skin, hair, and vaginal tissues healthy and also to enhance the production of beneficial prostaglandins, which aid in hormone production. Most women generally get sufficient amounts of omega-6 fatty acids, which are found in nuts, grains, vegetable oils, and meats from land animals. Omega-3 fatty acids are more difficult to come by and are critical for maintaining a healthful balance of prostaglandins as well as for maintaining optimal health. Foods that are good sources of omega-3 fatty acids include cold-water fish (such as salmon, trout, and mackerel), flaxseeds, flaxseed oil, and raw walnuts. Gamma linolenic acid (GLA) is also essential for the production of prostaglandins. Under ideal circumstances the body makes GLA from omega-6 fatty acids, but because many factors (including aging), interfere with the production of this important nutrient many women suffer from a deficiency. GLA is available in supplements in the form of evening primrose oil, black currant oil, and borage oil. Take enough capsules to equal 240 milligrams of GLA daily for three to six months, and then cut the dosage in half and continue taking the supplement indefinitely.

Diet is a primary factor in keeping blood-sugar levels consistent, which is critical for keeping tissues healthy and preventing degenerative disease. Maintaining stable blood-sugar levels also helps to prevent fatigue and depression. Eat frequent small meals and include a moderate amount of protein and healthful fats such as raw nuts and avocados. Avoid sugar and refined carbohydrates, which trigger the excessive production of insulin that causes blood-sugar instability. Dehydration is also a contributing factor to fatigue, so be sure to drink at least one quart of pure water daily. For more information on keeping blood-sugar levels balanced, see the information on hypoglycemia in Chapter 17.

Five Essential Herbs for Menopause

Herbs have been used for centuries by women in cultures throughout the world to ease the transition through menopause. Tonic herbs such as *Siberian ginseng* help to strengthen the reproductive and endocrine systems, balance hormones, and build vitality. They work gently over a period of months to replenish organs and glands and rebuild stores of vital energy. In general, it takes approximately three to six months to feel the full benefits of taking tonic herbs. The following herbs are especially beneficial during menopause.

Siberian ginseng *(Eleutherococcus senticosus)* is one of the best herbal energy tonics. It helps to strengthen the adrenal glands and also enhances immune function.

Licorice root *(Glycyrrhiza glabra)* contains compounds that are similar to the hormones produced by the adrenal glands. It has mild immediate energizing properties and helps to rebuild adrenal health. *If you have high blood pressure, do not use licorice root without first consulting your health practitioner.*

Vitex *(Vitex agnus castus)* helps to regulate the balance of estrogen and progesterone by stimulating the pituitary gland's secretion of FSH (follicle-stimulating hormone) and LH (luteinizing hormone).

Dong quai *(Angelica sinensis)* is referred to as the "Queen of Herbs" in Chinese medicine and is considered to be the primary tonic herb for women. It is especially beneficial during menopause because of its estrogen-like properties.

Black cohosh *(Cimifuga racemosa)* also has estrogen-like properties and helps to balance hormones. Clinical studies have shown that an extract of black cohosh is as effective as synthetic estrogen for relieving both the physical and psychological symptoms of menopause such as hot flashes, vaginal dryness, and depression, but without harmful side effects.

Make Your Own Hormone-Balancing Vitality Tonic

Virtually every woman who is perimenopausal or menopausal can benefit from taking an herbal tonic to strengthen and nourish her adrenal glands and reproductive organs. The following tonic will increase energy, restore a feeling of well-being and vitality, and help to ease the hormonal fluctuations that occur during menopause. For best results, take this tonic for at least three months. It can safely be taken indefinitely. If you have high blood pressure, leave the licorice root out of this formula.

Hormone-Balancing Vitality Tonic

1/2 ounce Siberian ginseng root
1/2 ounce vitex berries
1/2 ounce black cohosh root
1/4 ounce dong quai root
1/4 ounce licorice root
vodka

Follow the directions on page 10 for making an herbal extract. You can also buy prepared liquid herbal extracts and combine them in the same proportions. Take one teaspoon of the tonic in a small amount of warm water 3 times daily.

Exercise Away Menopausal Problems

Regular aerobic exercise is extremely important during the menopausal years. Not only does it help to relieve common symptoms such as hot flashes, but it strengthens the cardiovascular system and prevents osteoporosis. Aerobic exercise also decreases blood-cholesterol levels and blood pressure, improves circulation, increases energy and endurance, and helps you to maintain a healthful weight. In addition to the many physical benefits, exercise positively affects the mind and emotions by stimulating the production of endorphins, the body's natural mood-elevating substances. Plan for at least 30 minutes of aerobic exercise daily, in the form of walking, biking, dancing, or other activities that you enjoy.

Forms of meditative exercise such as yoga and tai chi are helpful during menopause for easing the tension that often accompanies this time of transition. The graceful, flowing movements encourage the free flow of energy and promote unity of the body, mind, and spirit. In addition, allowing time for a daily practice of inward focusing through meditation, journaling, or visualization creates the opportunity to access your deepest needs and desires and helps to bring balance into your life.

Cool Hot Flashes

Almost 80 percent of menopausal women experience hot flashes, sudden episodes of warmth that begin on the chest, neck, or face and spread throughout the body. Hot flashes are caused by the dilation of peripheral blood vessels, which raises skin temperature by several degrees. The skin becomes red and warm for a few seconds to a couple of minutes and is usually accompanied by sweating, which for some women can be profuse. As the flush of heat subsides, cold chills often follow as perspiration evaporates and cools the body. The intensity and frequency of hot flashes varies greatly, and while most women experience approximately one hot flash daily, some are troubled by numerous flashes throughout the day and night. I have friends who refer to their hot flashes as "power surges." This is a great example of choosing to see the physiological changes of menopause in a positive light! But even with a positive attitude, these fluctuations in body temperature can be extremely uncomfortable. Other symptoms that often accompany hot flashes include increased heart rate, heart palpitations, breathlessness, headache, dizziness, fatigue, insomnia, weakness, numbness of hands and arms, and itchy skin. Hot flashes that occur during the night disturb normal sleep patterns and can cause insomnia, fatigue, and irritability.

Although the exact reason for hot flashes is not known for certain, they appear to be caused by the natural decrease in estrogen and progesterone that occurs during menopause. The drop in hormones affects the pituitary and hypothalamus, the glands that regulate temperature. Hot flashes are often the first sign of menopause and appear to reflect the body's efforts to adjust to a different balance of hormones. They tend to begin while a woman is still having menstrual periods, and usually occur during the menstrual flow. Hot flashes typically cause the most discomfort during the first year or two of menopause and tend to subside as the body adapts to lower levels of estrogen. However, some women still experience hot flashes almost a decade after completing menopause.

Eating to Relieve Hot Flashes

Eating foods rich in phytoestrogens, especially soy foods, has been shown to decrease the intensity of hot flashes by helping to balance estrogen levels. Try to eat one or two servings of soy foods such as tofu, tempeh, and soy milk each day (see recipes in Appendix I for suggestions). Dietary supplements that help to relieve hot flashes include vitamin E and bioflavonoids. In clinical studies, vitamin E has been shown to reduce the incidence of hot flashes. Take 400 to 800 I.U.s of natural vitamin E in the form of d-alpha tocopherol daily. If you suffer from hypertension or diabetes, check with your doctor before taking large amounts of vitamin E. Bioflavonoids are found abundantly in citrus fruits, especially in the white inner rind and pulp. Bioflavonoids have phytoestrogenic activity and have been shown to markedly reduce the incidence of hot flashes. Eat one or two servings of fresh citrus fruits daily, including as much of the white inner peel as possible. In addition, take supplemental bioflavonoids combined with vitamin C, which helps to strengthen adrenal function. Take 1,000 units of vitamin C combined with bioflavonoids three times a day.

Herbal Relief for Hot Flashes

Herbs have been used for centuries by women to prevent and relieve hot flashes. Cool herbal teas can be sipped throughout the day to keep your body well-hydrated. Try fragrant herbs such as *chamomile, linden flower,* and *mint,* which make delicious teas and have a calming and soothing effect on the mind and body. Many herbs, such as *black cohosh* and the Chinese herb *dong quai,* are rich in phytoestrogens, plant estrogens which help to normalize hormone levels. Taking these herbs regularly helps to balance hormones and prevent hot flashes. The Hormone Balancing tonic on page 86 is excellent for relieving hot flashes when taken regularly.

A cup of *sage* tea is a time-honored remedy for relieving hot flashes, particularly those that occur at night. My friend Lisa was exhausted from hot flashes that woke her during the night and left her drenched in a pool of perspiration. She found that drinking a cup of the following tea every night before bed reduced the frequency and severity of her hot flashes.

Hot Flash Relief Tea

2 tablespoons garden sage
1 tablespoon motherwort
2 teaspoons anise seeds
2 cups water

Pour boiling water over herbs, cover, and let steep until cool. Strain, and drink one cup of cool tea before bed.

The aromatic oil that gives garden sage *(Salvia officinalis)* its characteristic scent and flavor has strong astringent properties that reduce perspiration by up to 50 percent. *Motherwort* is a wonderful herbal ally for menopausal women; it has relaxing properties and helps to calm the heart palpitations that often accompany middle-of-the-night hot flashes. *Anise seeds* are a source of phytoestrogens and add a pleasant sweetness to the tea that helps to soften the bitterness of the motherwort. Insomnia often accompanies hot flashes that occur at night. If you are troubled by sleeplessness, add to the formula one tablespoon of *passionflower,* a pleasant-tasting herb that has gentle relaxing properties.

Ease Hot Flashes with Aromatherapy

Relaxing baths ease physical and emotional tension and are a wonderful treat for relieving the discomfort of hot flashes. Avoid hot water, which can raise body temperature and trigger hot flashes. Draw a tub of tepid water, and add one cup of baking soda as a skin soother. Essential oils add fragrance and subtle healing properties. *Lavender, geranium, clary sage,* and *rose* essential oils all help to balance hormones and promote relaxation. Add 5 to 10 drops total of one or more essential oils to a tubful of water.

You can enjoy the cooling and relaxing benefits of aromatherapy throughout the day by carrying a spray bottle filled with a refreshing facial mist.

Cooling Aromatherapy Facial Mist

1/4 cup aloe vera juice
1/4 cup rosewater
5 drops rose or lavender essential oil

Combine ingredients in a glass spray bottle and shake well. Mist skin as often as desired.

Cool Hot Flashes Naturally

Simple measures can help to alleviate hot flashes. Avoid overheating your home or workplace, and dress in layers that make it easy to add or remove clothing as needed. Natural fibers such as silk and linen help to maintain a comfortable body temperature by allowing perspiration to evaporate quickly. Keep a small paper or bamboo fan handy for quick cooling during a hot flash. Natural-fiber bedding will help to keep you comfortable during the night. Use pure cotton or linen sheets, and instead of one heavy blanket or comforter, sleep with thin layers of cotton or wool blankets and a lightweight down comforter that can be added or removed as needed.

Emotional stress is often a trigger for hot flashes. Practices such as deep rhythmical breathing and meditation create a calm internal environment that keeps your body and emotions in balance. See Appendix II for suggestions for relaxation and meditation practices. You can also relieve emotional and physical tension with regular exercise such as a daily half-hour brisk walk. Avoid walking in the hot sun, though, because excessive heat can bring on a hot flash. During hot weather, walk in the early morning or evening. Other types of exercise that have a calming and cooling effect are swimming, tai chi, and yoga. The long, slow stretches of yoga and the gentle, flowing movements of tai chi are excellent for creating a deep sense of peace and relaxation and are wonderful practices for bringing the body and mind into harmony.

Relieve Vaginal Dryness

Many women find that the decrease in estrogen that occurs during menopause causes the vaginal lining to become thin and dry, which often causes burning and itching and makes sexual intercourse painful. The thinning and drying of the vaginal tissues also creates an environment that is hospitable to vaginal infections. For natural treatments for vaginal infections, see Chapter 6.

Taking hormone-regulating herbs such as the formula given on page 86 can help to thicken the vaginal lining. Herbs in the form of oils and salves can also be applied directly to the vaginal tissues to soothe and heal irritation. *Calendula* and *comfrey* salves are particularly helpful for vaginal dryness. My friend Ann virtually breezed through menopause without any symptoms except for severe vaginal dryness. She made a large batch of comfrey salve and began applying a small amount daily to her irritated vaginal tissues. Within days, her vaginal tissues healed. She continues to use the salve to prevent further problems. Calendula and comfrey both have skin-healing and antimicrobial properties that help to fight infection. In addition, comfrey contains allantoin, a natural compound that spurs the regeneration of healthy skin tissue. You can buy calendula and comfrey salves, or make your own with the recipe on page 11. Apply the salve once or twice daily as needed. Some women also find that vitamin E helps to heal irritated vaginal tissues. Try inserting a 1,000-I.U. vitamin E gelatin capsule into the vagina every night before bed. The gelatin will dissolve at body temperature, allowing the vitamin E to coat the vaginal tissues.

To protect delicate vaginal tissues, stay away from anything that tends to dry the mucous membranes, including harsh soaps, bubble baths, douches, and feminine-hygiene sprays. Also avoid taking antihistamines and diuretics, because they deplete the body tissues of fluids, and drink at least one quart of water daily. To prevent vaginal irritation, wear natural-fiber clothing, which allows air to circulate and decreases the risk of vaginal infection. Regular sexual activity keeps the vaginal tissues healthy by increasing blood flow and stimulating natural lubrication. If you need extra lubrication during sexual intercourse, use a healing oil such as calendula oil (see recipe page 11).

Overcome Urinary Problems

The tissue thinning that occurs during menopause affects not only the vaginal tissues but also the tissues of the urinary tract. As with the vaginal mucous membranes, the lining of the urethra becomes thinner and less elastic after menopause. This tissue thinning increases the likelihood of urinary tract infections and can also cause problems with urinary incontinence (for more information on urinary tract infections, see Chapter 5). Urinary incontinence is a distressing problem that manifests as the need to urinate more frequently with varying degrees of loss of bladder control. Urine leakage is often triggered by coughing, sneezing, or laughing.

The Hormone Balancing formula on page 86 is helpful for restoring the thickness of the urinary tract tissues. To help to heal irritated urinary tract membranes, drink herbal teas from soothing herbs such as *marshmallow root,* which contains a large amount of mucilage, a natural plant sugar that helps to relieve inflammation. To regain control over the urinary tract muscles and prevent incontinence, practice Kegel exercises (named for the doctor who developed them). These exercises take only a few minutes and are very effective. You can perform them standing, sitting, or lying down, and you can practice anywhere and anytime that is convenient for you. These exercises are great for times when you don't have anything better to do—for example, while you are standing in line or sitting at a traffic light. No one will ever know what you are doing. The important thing is to practice consistently to strengthen the muscles.

Here's how to practice Kegels: First, contract the pubococcygeus (PC) muscle, the same muscle that you would use to stop urinating in midstream. Repeat the contraction ten times, holding each contraction for three seconds, and relaxing for three seconds between contractions. Now squeeze the PC muscle, but this time release it as quickly as possible. Repeat this fluttering contraction ten times. Repeat the entire sequence three times a day, and increase the number of repetitions as you are able until you build up to three sets of 20 contractions of both exercises three times daily.

Arrest Heavy Bleeding

Heavy menstrual bleeding is common as a woman approaches menopause. As hormone levels begin to shift and there is an excess of estrogen in relation to progesterone, a woman typically will have periods that are closer together with more profuse bleeding. Any type of abnormally heavy bleeding should be evaluated by your doctor to rule out problems such as fibroids, endometriosis, or uterine cancer. If you do have any of these conditions, refer to the chapters on these topics for specific recommendations.

Fatigue is often a problem with heavy bleeding because of blood and iron loss. Drink three cups daily of a nutrient-rich herbal tea such as *nettle* to help build healthy red-blood cells. Nettle is high in iron and other minerals and makes a pleasant tasting tea. Use two teaspoons of nettle per cup of water and follow the directions on page 9 for making an herbal infusion. For an extra boost of iron, take *yellow dock root* extract, an herb that is exceptionally rich in easily assimilable iron. You can drink yellow dock root tea, but the flavor is bitter and it doesn't make a tasty beverage. (If you want to make a tea, follow the directions on page 9 for making an herbal decoction.) Take one-half teaspoon of yellow dock root liquid extract or two capsules twice a day until blood-iron levels return to normal. You can also make your own yellow dock root extract by following the recipe on page 10 for making extracts.

Ease Emotional Unrest

Shifting hormones and the life changes that commonly occur during midlife can make menopause a time of emotional unrest. Many women feel confused and distressed by the emotional and physical upheavals they are experiencing, and it's not uncommon to feel anxiety, depression, and irritability during this time of great change. The Western view of menopause has certainly not been supportive; instead, it has been detrimental and demeaning to women. Our culture's undue emphasis on youth and physical attractiveness has caused many women to fear menopause, as they associate the loss of youth and fertility with diminished sexual desirability and attractiveness. Fortunately, this narrow and harmful viewpoint is changing as women are refusing to continue accepting the cultural stereotypes. It is up to us, as women, to actively change these negative images that our culture has created. We must cultivate a sense of value for ourselves and for each other that is not based on externals, but rather is rooted in a reverence for life and an appreciation of the individual uniqueness of each of us.

It is time to stop accepting the negative assumptions that our culture has made about aging. The truth is that women who have developed a strong sense of self and who find gratification in family, friends, work, and other interests report great satisfaction in life and adjust much more easily to the actual physical changes that occur during menopause. Midlife can be a wonderful opportunity to cultivate interests that bring meaning to your life. You may decide to go back to school, change careers, volunteer your time to help others, express yourself creatively, or become active in a cause that matters to you. Whatever path you choose, allow yourself time to reflect on what is meaningful to you at this time in your life. Many women find it helpful to share their feelings about this important life passage with friends, in women's groups, or in therapy. Keeping a journal can be a healing process that helps you to access your inner self. Honor your feelings, your thoughts, and your dreams in the process of creating your present and future.

It is true that shifting hormones affect your emotional state, and there are many ways of naturally helping to bring your emotions into balance. The brain produces compounds called endorphins, natural chemicals that are associated with feelings of well-being. The drop in estrogen and progesterone levels that occurs during menopause is accompanied by a decrease in endorphins, which can trigger feelings of depression or anxiety. You can significantly increase your body's production of endorphins through pleasurable activities such as massage, exercise, meditation, and sex. Virtually anything you do that makes you feel good triggers the release of endorphins. Spend time in activities that connect you with nature, such as gardening, hiking, or simply relaxing outdoors. Allow time for creative pursuits such as writing, art, or music—try something new that intrigues you.

Herbs can be a wonderful support during times of emotional stress, depression, or anxiety. For mild emotional tension, drink teas made from *chamomile, lemon balm,* or *linden flower. St. John's wort* is excellent for mild to moderate depression and is as effective as the pharmaceutical antidepressants that are commonly prescribed, but without the unpleasant side effects. For anxiety, take *kava kava,* a powerful yet safe herb from Polynesia that has an immediate relaxing effect. For a more thorough discussion of herbs and other natural approaches for treating anxiety and depression, see Chapters 13 and 14.

Chapter 11

Enhance Your Sexual Vitality

A woman's sexuality is an outward manifestation of the creativity and passion of her inner self and can be an avenue for joyful self-expression and self-renewal. Some women fear that menopause signals the end of their sexuality. This is especially true if hormonal changes are causing fatigue or vaginal changes that make sex painful. Menopause does end your fertile years, but it does not portend the demise of sexual and sensual pleasure. Basically, if you enjoyed sex before menopause, then you will enjoy it afterwards. In fact, many women find that they have much more satisfying sex after menopause. This is because the hormonal changes that occur during menopause serve to enhance, not diminish, sexual responsiveness. A woman's sexual arousal is dependent on testosterone (although testosterone is primarily a male hormone, women also have small amounts). After menopause, when estrogen and progesterone levels drop, there is a proportionately greater amount of testosterone, which stimulates a greater enjoyment of sex.

While these hormonal changes have a positive effect on sexuality, during the time that your body is adjusting to different levels of hormones you may feel fatigued and not particularly interested in sex, especially if you are suffering from hot flashes and other symptoms that deplete your energy. Declining estrogen levels may also cause vaginal dryness and thinning, which can make sexual intercourse painful. These symptoms can be managed with natural remedies, and most women find that their sexual interest returns as their body adjusts to a new and different hormone balance.

In addition to the physiological changes in your body, your personal beliefs about sex and aging have a profound influence on how you feel about sexuality and sensuality. This can be a wonderful time for exploring your sensuality and for discovering what feels good to you. Many women find that menopause brings new opportunities for sexual and sensual exploration. They enjoy the freedom from worrying about pregnancy, birth control, and monthly bleeding, and may also have more leisure time for sexual play. Healthy sexuality can bring love, intimacy, and great sensual pleasure to life, and it is worth cultivating.

Unfortunately, the Western view of sexuality has primarily focused on sex for procreation and has labeled eroticism and sensuality as sinful. Even though much has changed in the past few decades, there is still an uncomfortableness with sensual and sexual pleasure that permeates our society. The ancient Eastern view of sex was much healthier. They taught that sex is a gift that enhances intimacy and pleasure and that healthy sex is an important means for cultivating life energy, healing, and self-knowledge. The primary focus is not on orgasm, but on giving and receiving sensual pleasure. In other words, the journey is much more important than the destination. You can cultivate sexual and sensual pleasure through meditative exercises, breathing techniques, and herbs, foods, and essential oils that enhance your experience of sensuality.

Exercises for Increasing Sexual Energy

Exercise in general is important for sexual vitality because it builds endurance, strength, and flexibility. Your body thrives on movement, and physical activity helps to keep your body balanced and your energy flowing. The more physically fit you are, the more sex-

ual energy you will have. Vigorous exercise also stimulates the production of endorphins, the natural brain chemicals that have an
uplifting effect on your emotions. However, avoid overexercising,
which can cause fatigue and diminish your sexual vitality. Moderate
daily exercise, such as brisk walking, dancing, or bicycling, that
makes you feel energized, but not depleted, is best. Another benefit of regular exercise is that it helps you feel good about your body,
which heightens feelings of sensuality.

To specifically enhance sexual pleasure, practice the Kegel
exercises, which strengthen the pubococcygeus (PC) muscle, the
muscle that extends from the pubic bone to the coccyx (tailbone)
and is part of the musculature that supports the internal pelvic
organs. Like any other muscle, the PC muscle loses tone if it is not
exercised. Diminished vaginal sensitivity and lessened sexual pleasure can result from lack of muscle tone, as can urinary incontinence
and uterine prolapse. These exercises were originally created to help
women who were suffering from urinary incontinence by strengthening the muscle that controls urine flow. Women practicing these
exercises experienced wonderful results—and not just with urinary
control. They reported increased pleasure during sex and better and
stronger orgasms. Kegel exercises strengthen the same muscles that
contract during orgasm, bring increased circulation to the genitals,
improve vaginal tissue tone, and help to increase sexual enjoyment
for you and your partner. With regular exercise of the PC muscle, the
entire pelvic region becomes healthier.

To practice Kegels, contract the muscle that you would use to
stop urinating in midstream. Hold the contraction for a count of three,
and then release for a count of three. Repeat this ten times. Now
rapidly contract and release the same muscle ten times as quickly as
you can. Repeat ten times. You can also practice Kegels lying down,
which strengthens both the PC muscle and the internal organs. Lie on
your back with your knees bent and your feet flat on the floor. Lift
your pelvis a couple of inches off the floor and contract the PC muscle. Practice the sequence of Kegel exercises as described.

While the focus of Kegel exercises is on enhancing sexuality
through improving muscle tone, you may also wish to explore
ancient Eastern practices that concentrate on enhancing energy
flow. Yoga and tai chi are two meditative, flowing forms of exercise
that promote the free flow of energy throughout the body and help
to relieve stagnation in the pelvic area. Blocked energy can cause

lack of sexual interest or difficulty in feeling sexual pleasure. More esoteric exercises come from ancient Taoist practices that focus on using the mind and breathing techniques for enhancing energy flow and building sexual energy. Thousands of years ago, the Taoists created an elaborate system of longevity that included the careful cultivation of sexual energy. They taught that energy flows throughout the body in channels called meridians and created specific exercises to increase energy flow and improve the health of the internal organs. Making love in this way returns sexual energy to the endocrine glands, which nourishes them and encourages the production of sex hormones.

Ancient Wisdom for Sexual Pleasure

A three-part exercise based on ancient Taoist practices can help you build sexual energy and awareness while strengthening your sexual organs. First, sit in a comfortable position. Close your eyes and pay attention to the flow of your breath as it enters and leaves your body. As you inhale, expand your abdomen, and as you exhale, draw your abdomen in gently toward your spine. For more specific instructions in learning the practice of deep abdominal breathing, refer to the exercises in Appendix II. Breathe rhythmically in this way for several minutes. Regulating your breathing calms your mind, sharpens your senses, and increases your ability to focus your attention, all of which contribute to heightened body awareness.

Second, when you feel relaxed, change the flow of your breathing so that as you inhale, you draw your abdomen in toward your spine, and as you exhale, you gently expand your abdomen. This reverse breathing generates energy in the pelvic area. Continue breathing in this way throughout the remainder of this exercise.

The third part of this exercise strengthens the pubococcygeus muscle, the same muscle that you concentrate on in the Kegel exercises. To strengthen the PC muscle, tighten the muscles of your vagina and anus as though you are trying to close both openings, draw them up toward your navel, and then relax. Coordinate the muscle contractions with your breathing so that when you inhale and draw your abdomen in, you are contracting your vagina and anus, and when you exhale, you are releasing your abdomen and the muscles of your vagina and anus. Practice this meditative breathing exercise for ten minutes daily to strengthen your internal muscles and build sexual energy.

For a simple exercise that concentrates energy in the pelvis and enhances sexual energy, stand in a comfortable position with your feet hip-width apart and your knees relaxed. Take a couple of slow, deep breaths to relax, inhaling and exhaling in an easy rhythm. Close your eyes, and rub your palms briskly together until you generate warmth in your hands. When your hands feel warm, briskly rub your palms over your kidney area (your low mid-back on either side of your spine) for 15 to 30 seconds. Rub your hands together again for a few seconds to generate energy in your palms, and then immediately place your palms over your lower abdomen for 30 seconds. As you feel the warmth from your hands, imagine that energy is circulating throughout your pelvis, healing and energizing your sexual organs.

Rub your hands briskly together again, and place your palms over your kidneys with your fingers pointing down. Slowly begin to rotate your hips in a small clockwise circle (imagine that you are drawing a circle on the floor) while keeping your upper body still. Inhale as you rotate your hips to the rear, and exhale as you circle forward. Repeat this circular movement 25 times in a clockwise direction, and then repeat 25 circles to the left.

Foods That Strengthen Sexual Vitality

Throughout the centuries people have sought out foods with aphrodisiacal powers and have proclaimed everything from oysters and figs to bird's-nest soup and rhinoceros horns as sexual stimulants. While there is some truth to certain foods strengthening sexual energy (oysters, for example, are extremely rich in zinc, a critical nutrient for the reproductive organs), the best approach to ensure sexual vitality is to eat a balanced whole-foods diet. Choose a varied diet centered around plenty of fresh vegetables and fruits, lean proteins such as fish and poultry, legumes, and whole grains. To enhance the production of prostaglandins, hormone-like substances that are important for sexual response, be sure to include foods rich in essential fatty acids, particularly omega-3 fatty acids, found in cold-water fish (salmon, sardines, mackerel), flaxseeds, flaxseed oil, and walnuts. Supplements of another essential fatty acid called gamma linolenic acid (GLA) are also helpful for building prostaglandins.

Take between 120 and 240 milligrams of GLA daily in the form of evening primrose, borage, or black currant seed oil. Avoid foods that cause energy depletion, especially caffeine, sugar, alcohol, high-fat foods, and processed foods. Pay attention to your adrenal glands, which help to provide sexual vitality, and follow the guidelines on page 82 for strengthening your adrenal function. To ensure that you are getting all of the nutrients necessary for optimal health, take a high-potency vitamin-and-mineral supplement daily.

In Chinese medicine, foods are used to strengthen the *kidney chi,* or *essence,* which is believed to govern sexual vitality and long-term health. Some of the symptoms of weakened essence include fatigue, sore lower back, and loss of sexual interest. Foods that restore essence include sesame seeds, black beans, walnuts, shrimp, salmon, and chicken. Chinese herbs that restore essence such as *cooked rehmannia root, dioscorea, cornus,* and *lycii* are cooked into soups with essence-replenishing foods and eaten one or more times a week. Cooked rehmannia root is a sticky, smoky-sweet dark-black root, cornus is a mildly tart fruit, dioscorea is a soft, starchy tuber, and lycii is a small, sweet-tart red berry. All are readily available in Chinese herb stores, and also by mail order (see Resources, page 338). Try the following recipe for a delicious soup that will help to restore and maintain sexual vitality.

Essence-Replenishing Soup

7 cups chicken stock
1 ounce cooked rehmannia root
1 ounce dioscorea rhizome
1/2 ounce cornus fruit
1/2 ounce lycii berries
1 inch fresh ginger root, minced
1/2 cup cooked diced chicken
1/2 cup carrots, thinly sliced
1/2 cup scallions, thinly sliced
1/4 teaspoon sea salt
tamari and toasted sesame oil

(continued)

- *Break the dioscorea into 1/2-inch pieces.*

- *Simmer the rehmannia, dioscorea, cornus, lycii, and ginger in the chicken stock in a covered pot for one and 1/2 hours.*

- *Add the chicken, carrots, and sea salt, and simmer for an additional 15 minutes.*

- *Add the scallions and season with tamari (natural soy sauce) and a few drops of toasted sesame oil to taste.*

Herbs for Sexual Enhancement

A variety of different herbs can be used to enhance sexuality. Some herbs, such as *ginseng* and *dong quai,* help to tonify and strengthen the endocrine system and the reproductive organs. When taken over a period of several months, they increase overall vitality and can be considered sexual tonics. Other herbs, such as *damiana,* can be considered aphrodisiacs, because they heighten the sensitivity of the sexual organs and are usually taken in preparation for lovemaking. The following herbs are some of the most important for enhancing sexuality.

American ginseng *(Panax quinquefolius)* is a rejuvenative tonic that increases overall well-being and endurance. It is most effective when taken over a period of several months.

Donq quai *(Angelica sinensis)* is considered in Chinese medicine to be the premier tonic herb for women. It helps to bring hormones into balance and regulates the entire reproductive system.

Damiana *(Turnera diffusa)* grows in the desert areas of Mexico and the southwestern United States. It contains a volatile oil that gently stimulates the genitourinary tract when it is excreted, which acts to enhance sexual arousal. It also has mild euphoric and muscle-relaxing properties. Damiana has been used for centuries by Mexican women who traditionally drink a cup of damiana tea before lovemaking.

Aphrodisiac Tea

2 tablespoons damiana leaves

1 teaspoon rose petals

1 teaspoon anise seeds

1 teaspoon mint leaves

2 cups water

Pour water over herbs, cover, and steep for 10 minutes. Strain, sweeten if desired, and drink 1 or 2 cups one hour before love-making.

The following herbal formula is a long-term energy builder for enhancing sexual vitality. It is best taken for at least three months or longer. Do not take this formula during your menstrual cycle, because dong quai can stimulate bleeding.

Sexual-Vitality Formula

1 ounce dong-quai root (whole or sliced)

1 ounce American ginseng root (whole)

2 ounces vitex berries, crushed

2 ounces damiana leaves

4 vanilla beans, split

1 nutmeg, grated

brandy

1 cup honey

- *Place herbs in a glass container with a tight-fitting lid and add enough brandy to cover the herbs by three inches.*

- *Cover tightly, and store in a cool, dark place for 3 weeks. Give the jar a gentle shake every day or two to keep the herbs from settling.*

(continued)

- *After 3 weeks, strain out the herbs, reserving the ginseng and dong quai. Discard the other herbs.*

- *Warm the honey slightly to liquefy it and add it to the herbal-brandy mixture. Pour into a glass bottle, and return the reserved ginseng and dong quai to the bottle.*

- *Take one teaspoon twice daily.*

Cultivating Your Sensuality

We are sensual beings and are affected on conscious and subconscious levels by the sounds, scents, colors, sensations, and tastes that surround us. In addition to exercises, foods, and herbs that build sexual vitality, you can enhance your sexuality with essential oils, massage, baths, and other pleasures that awaken your sensuality. Taking the time for a special meditation or bath, or making the effort to prepare an herbal aphrodisiac affirms your desire to nourish your sexuality, and it is this desire that is perhaps the most potent aphrodisiac of all. Don't confine your sensual enjoyment only to lovemaking, but surround yourself with what brings you pleasure.

Take the time to create an environment that nourishes your senses, choosing colors, fabrics, music, and fragrances that you find sensually pleasing. Creating an atmosphere conducive to sensuality and lovemaking is like preparing for a celebration. The more you put into it, the more pleasure you are likely to get out of it. Touch is extremely important to sensual and sexual pleasure, and not just touch that is focused on the genitals. Massage is a wonderful way of awakening the senses, and fragrant essential oils add additional pleasure.

Essential Oils as Aphrodisiacs

Scent has a powerful effect on the mind and the body and can greatly enhance sensual enjoyment. The sense of smell is controlled by the limbic system, the part of the brain that is the center for emotions, memories, and sexuality. Because fragrance directly influences the limbic part of the brain, many essential oils have long been valued as aphrodisiacs.

Rose is especially beneficial for women. It helps to balance hormones, has a tonic effect on the reproductive organs, and enhances sexuality. Psychologically, rose is uplifting and helps to restore a woman's connection to her femininity.

Sandalwood induces a state of calmness and serenity and relieves nervous tension. It is considered a sexual restorative for both women and men and has a rich, deep, woodsy-sweet scent.

Ylang-ylang is deeply relaxing, exotic, and sensuous. It has a rich, intensely sweet floral fragrance that can be overpowering in excess. Use it in very small quantities—two or three drops at most in a bath.

Patchouli has been used for thousands of years as a sexual stimulant. It also relieves nervous exhaustion. This ancient fragrance has a rich, deep, earthy, herbaceous scent.

Jasmine relieves nervous tension, has mild euphoric properties, and is said to restore sexual confidence. It has an exotic, warm, fruity-floral fragrance.

Clary sage helps to balance hormones. It has sedative, almost euphoric properties and relieves emotional tension that can interfere with sexuality. It has a deep, sweet, herbaceous fragrance.

Sensual-Pleasures Massage Oil

3 ounces almond oil

1 ounce jojoba oil

20 drops sandalwood essential oil

10 drops rose essential oil

5 drops clary sage essential oil

Combine almond oil, jojoba oil, and essential oils in a dark glass bottle. Cap tightly, shake well, and store in a cool, dark place.

Exotic Herbal Bath

1 cup Epsom salts
1 cup baking soda
5 drops sandalwood essential oil
2 drops rose essential oil
2 drops ylang-ylang essential oil
handful of rose petals

- *Draw a tubful of comfortably warm water, light a candle, and put on music that you find sensual and relaxing.*

- *While the water is running, add the Epsom salts (a muscle relaxant) and baking soda (a skin softener) to the tub.*

- *After the tub has filled, add the essential oils, mixing the oils into the bathwater with your hand.*

- *Toss in the rose petals, and enter the tub for a relaxing soak.*

Chapter 12

Conquer Fatigue and Increase Your Energy

Do you feel vital and energetic most of the time, or like many women, are you chronically fatigued? If you're tired more often than you'd like to be, you're not alone. Fatigue is the number one health complaint, and although it can be a symptom of virtually any physical or emotional disorder, it is most often caused by poor diet, stress, vitamin and mineral deficiencies, anemia, depression, low-thyroid function, and hypoglycemia. The physiological changes that occur at menopause are also a prime cause of fatigue because hormonal shifts affect energy levels. When you feel tired, your body is giving you a clear message that it's time to stop and take time for rest and rejuvenation.

Your energy levels are a direct result of how well you nurture yourself physically and emotionally. Think of your energy stores as you do your bank account—if you take out more than you put in, you end up with a deficit. If you pay attention to regularly replenishing your energy, you will have the vitality to sustain you not only today, but for the decades of life that lie ahead. Vitality at midlife and beyond is directly related to how well you care for your body, mind, and spirit. Physical vitality can be strengthened with a healthful diet, nutritional supplements, exercise, rest, and herbal tonics that support the endocrine system. On a psychological and spiritual level, vitality comes from doing what you enjoy—cultivating interests and activities that make you look forward to getting up in the morning. For many women, midlife is a time of awakening to new possibilities. In order to fully enjoy the second half of your life, you must pay attention to nourishing your life energy, which manifests as vitality.

Toxins: A Common Cause of Fatigue

In your quest for more energy, it's important to look first at what is draining your vitality. One of the primary underlying causes of fatigue is the accumulation of toxic substances in the body. We are continually assaulted by toxins, both externally and internally. Not only do we take in toxins through inhaling, ingesting, and coming into physical contact with the thousands of chemicals that taint our environment, food, and water, but our bodies also create toxins as a natural by-product of everyday metabolic functions. For example, intestinal bacteria generate waste products that have to be eliminated, and the process of digesting protein creates nitrogen wastes that are poisonous if they are not excreted by the kidneys. Basically, a toxin is any substance that irritates the cells and interferes with the normal functioning of the body. Toxicity and fatigue occur when your body is exposed to large quantities of toxins, or when your normal pathways of detoxification—your liver, large intestine, kidneys, lungs, skin, and lymphatic system—are not functioning up to par.

When your body is functioning optimally, it has a variety of built-in controls for handing toxins. It either eliminates the offending substance, or it transforms it into a less harmful compound. Our bodies evolved with the ability to neutralize and eliminate toxins, but were not designed to handle the large amounts of harmful chemicals that we now encounter on a daily basis. The load of poisons we are exposed to overwhelms the organs of detoxification, and the resultant accumulation of toxins further impedes healthy organ functioning. For vitality and well-being, you need to support your organs of detoxification by reducing your exposure to toxins, eating a healthful diet low in food stressors, and by taking herbs and supplements that help your body to detoxify.

How to Help Your Body Detoxify

The following steps will help you reduce your exposure to toxic substances, which eases the burden on your body's organs of detoxification.

- Buy organically grown food (or grow your own) to limit your exposure to pesticides, herbicides, and other dangerous agricultural chemicals.
- Avoid dietary stressors such as caffeine, sugar, alcohol, and processed foods.
- Don't smoke, and avoid exposure to secondhand smoke.
- Eliminate unhealthful fats such as hydrogenated fats, polyunsaturated oils, and fried foods.
- Use filtered or spring water to avoid exposure to chlorine and other poisonous chemicals.
- Seek natural alternatives to over-the-counter and prescription drugs.
- Use natural, nontoxic alternatives to household and garden chemicals.
- Use air filters if necessary to improve the air quality in your home and at work.

Herbs for Detoxification

Herbs have been used for centuries for cleansing and detoxification. All traditional healing systems, including the Ayurvedic, Chinese, and European herbal traditions, have regarded detoxification as essential for health. Stringent methods of detoxification, such as prolonged fasting, can deplete your energy. But the regular use of gentle cleansing herbs helps to eliminate the toxins that diminish energy and assists in bringing your body into balance. An herbal cleansing formula can be used one or more times a year to keep your body in optimal health. Cleansing herbs stimulate the elimination of wastes, increase urination, encourage perspiration, stimulate circulation, enhance immune functioning, and improve digestion. A balanced herbal cleansing formula supports each organ system that is involved in detoxification—the large intestine, liver, kidneys, lymphatic system, skin, and lungs.

The following herbal tea blend is excellent for gently stimulating detoxification. Drink this tea for two to three weeks in the early spring and fall.

Herbal Cleansing Tea

1 teaspoon burdock root
1 teaspoon echinacea root
1 teaspoon dandelion root
1 teaspoon licorice root
1 teaspoon ginger root
1 teaspoon nettle
1 teaspoon red clover
4 cups water

Combine burdock, echinacea, dandelion, licorice, and ginger with water. Bring to a boil in a covered pot over medium heat, reduce heat, and simmer gently for 15 minutes. Remove from heat, add nettle and red clover, cover, and steep for 15 minutes. Strain, and drink 3 to 4 cups daily.

Eating to Restore Vitality

At midlife, you may notice that you can't get by with the same things that you could when you were in your twenties or thirties. As we age, our bodies are not as resilient as they once were. On a physical level, vitality is determined by what we choose to eat and by what we choose to *not* eat. Caffeine, sugar, and alcohol are the most common and seductive energy zappers. Many women rely on caffeine and sugar for energy to get through the day, and then use alcohol at night for relaxation. Grabbing a cup of coffee, a cola, or a sugary snack provides a jolt of energy, but it ultimately weakens your organs and glands and creates a deeper level of fatigue.

Caffeine is a powerful stimulant that temporarily provides a feeling of energy and alertness, but at a significant cost to your health. By stimulating your adrenal glands, caffeine keeps your body in a perpetual state of arousal and causes nervousness, anxiety, and insomnia. It also robs your body of essential nutrients, including potassium, magnesium, calcium, and B-complex vitamins. When you take in caffeine, you are depleting your body of the nutrients it needs to maintain a stable mood and good energy level.

Sugar in any form—including honey, maple syrup, and molasses—is quickly absorbed into your bloodstream, where it provides an energy rush to your cells. This energy is short-lived, however. Increased sugar in the bloodstream overstimulates the pancreas and adrenal glands and causes large amounts of insulin to be released, which sharply drops blood-sugar levels. Blood sugar imbalances such as hypoglycemia and diabetes often appear after the age of 40 because the adrenal glands and pancreas have lost their resiliency after years of trying to balance the effects of a high-sugar diet. Sugar also depletes nutrient reserves, especially B-vitamins and minerals, because it requires additional vitamins and minerals to be metabolized.

Alcohol is metabolized in much the same way as sugar, and because it has little nutritional value, it drains vitamins and minerals from body reserves. In addition, alcohol has toxic effects on the nervous system and the liver. It interferes with the liver's ability to metabolize hormones efficiently and worsens the hormonal fluctuations that occur in the perimenopausal and menopausal years. Because the negative effects of these commonly accepted stimulants start to show up in earnest at midlife, you have to be more consistent about eating a healthful, nutrient-rich diet if you want to feel as energetic as possible. Follow the dietary suggestions in Chapter 26, and avoid caffeine, sugar, and alcohol as best you can. It's not realistic nor is it necessary for most women to follow an unnecessarily restrictive, spartan regime, but if you use caffeine, sugar, or alcohol, make them occasional treats instead of a part of your daily diet.

Many women find it helpful to eat several small meals throughout the day instead of two or three larger meals. This helps to keep energy levels balanced, particularly if you choose healthful foods that provide sustained energy. Including a bit of protein or fat makes a snack satisfying—try an apple with a few almonds, yogurt with berries and walnuts, or whole-grain crackers with almond butter and carrot sticks. For beverages, drink green tea or herbal teas instead of coffee or other caffeinated drinks. Green tea has a mild energizing effect but does not stress the adrenal glands, and because it contains potent antioxidant compounds it has many health-protective benefits. Keep intensely sweet desserts to a minimum, and as often as possible, use fresh fruit to satisfy your sweet tooth.

Anemia can cause fatigue, and women who bleed heavily in the perimenopausal years are particularly at risk. Iron-rich foods or supplements can easily relieve anemia, but do not take supplemental iron without first having a blood test to make sure that you are iron deficient. Iron can accumulate in the body to dangerous levels and is a causative factor in heart disease and cancer. If you are anemic, include more foods in your diet that are good sources of iron, such as pumpkin seeds, lentils, spinach, raisins, and green peas. Animal foods such as chicken, eggs, and salmon contain less iron than many vegetables, but the iron is better absorbed.

To ensure that you are getting all of the vitamins and minerals necessary for optimal health, take a high-potency multivitamin-and-mineral supplement that contains 50 to 100 milligrams of the B-complex vitamins, which are especially important for energy. Potassium is also a critical nutrient for relieving fatigue, but supplements are unnecessary as long as you are eating an abundance of fresh fruits and vegetables. In addition to eating foods and taking supplements that supply your body with the nutrients it needs to build and sustain energy, be sure to drink plenty of pure water throughout the day. Strive for about eight glasses of filtered or spring water or herbal teas—fluids keep you from becoming dehydrated, which is a common and often unrecognized cause of fatigue.

Herbal Tonics for Energy Enhancement

For centuries, tonic herbs have been highly valued in Chinese medicine for their ability to preserve and restore vitality. These herbs are meant to be taken on a long-term basis—think of them as concentrated foods that directly nourish your deep stores of life energy. Choose one and try it for a couple of months to judge its effects. If you like it, you can continue taking it, or you can alternate various energy-building tonics every couple of months.

Ginseng *(Panax ginseng* and *Panax quinquefolium)* is said to replace lost *chi,* or life energy, and numerous research studies support its reputation as a restorative tonic. Ginseng helps the body adapt more easily to physical and emotional stressors by strengthening the function of the adrenal glands. Ginseng can sometimes cause overstimulation, with symptoms such as headaches or irritability. If this occurs, cut back on the amount you are taking and use American ginseng *(Panax quinquefolium)* because it is less stimulating than the Chinese variety. Ginseng is best used cyclically to prevent the problem of overstimulation—take it for two weeks, and then take a two-week break before resuming the dosage. For best results, buy an extract standardized for ginsenosides, which are considered to be the active compounds. Ginseng supplements vary widely in concentration—follow the manufacturer's instructions and decrease the dosage if necessary.

Ho shou wu *(Polygonum multiflorum)* also called fo-ti, is a Chinese herb that is similar to ginseng in its effects, but milder. It is considered to be a beneficial tonic for the reproductive organs, liver, and kidneys, all of which are critical for energy and vitality. Ho shou wu is also a tonic for the thyroid gland, which helps to regulate metabolism and energy. Because ho shou wu is not an immediate energizer, you need to take it over a long period of time (usually at least a couple of months) to feel the effects. Take one-half teaspoon of liquid extract two to three times daily in a small amount of warm water.

Siberian ginseng *(Eleutherococcus senticosus),* although not a true ginseng, has very similar properties and is a whole-body tonic that helps to restore healthy adrenal functioning. It significantly increases energy for both physical and mental tasks and bolsters resistance to stress. Taking Siberian ginseng regularly helps to increase both physical and psychological well-being. Take 250 milligrams two times a day of an extract standardized for eleutherosides, which are considered to be the active ingredient. For best results, take Siberian ginseng in cycles of two months, followed by a two-week break before resuming the dosage.

Exercise to Build Vitality

Although exercising may be the last thing you feel like doing when you are tired, regular exercise is essential for building vitality. Moderate aerobic exercise stimulates circulation and metabolism, improves digestion and lymphatic function, and infuses your body with fresh oxygen, which ensures the healthy functioning of every organ, gland, and cell in your body. When your cells are deprived of oxygen, fatigue quickly results. While a lack of exercise weakens your body and makes you feel sluggish, regular exercise increases your energy and endurance. But don't try to do too much too quickly, or you may find exercise tiring instead of energizing. Set realistic goals, and choose an activity that you find pleasurable. Walking is an ideal form of exercise—it's convenient, you can do it almost anywhere, and you can adjust your workout to your level of fitness. If you have not been exercising regularly, begin with a 15-minute walk every other day. Gradually increase your workout until you are walking a minimum of 30 minutes five days a week. If you are exercising the right amount for your level of fitness, you should feel energized after exercising, not exhausted.

Yoga and tai chi are excellent forms of exercise to supplement a walking program. Both help to build stores of vitality by improving breathing, oxygenating cells, increasing circulation, stretching the muscles, enhancing the function of organs and glands, and relieving physical tension. In addition, the slow, meditative movements of yoga and tai chi help to calm the mind and emotions. Try the following yoga exercises to build energy. Practice them ten minutes a day in the morning or in the afternoon.

CHEST EXPANDER

- Stand with your spine comfortably straight and your feet hip-width apart. Interlock your fingers behind your lower back, resting your hands on your buttocks.
- Inhale, and raise your arms behind you as high as you comfortably can, keeping your fingers interlocked. Keep your shoulders relaxed.
- Exhale, and lower your arms, again resting your hands on your buttocks. Repeat several times.

STANDING FORWARD BEND

- Stand with your feet a few inches apart and your back straight. Inhale, and raise your arms over your head, stretching upward.

- Exhale, and slowly bend from the waist, touching the floor or clasping your ankles, calves, or knees (whichever you can comfortably reach). Keep your legs straight but don't lock your knees. Hold for five seconds, breathing normally.

- Inhale as you slowly roll up to a standing position. Repeat two more times.

Lifestyle Suggestions to Increase Energy

- **Learn to manage stress.** Emotional tension is a tremendous contributing factor to fatigue because stress overworks the adrenal glands, which are critical for maintaining energy. It's not realistic to strive for a life without stress. A life without challenge would be boring, and some feelings of stress are normal in response to change or conflict. What's important is how you handle stress, and how much you allow it to affect your life and your health. If you frequently feel stressed, follow the suggestions in Chapter 13 to help you defuse the tension and anxiety that are sapping your energy.

- **Stop working too hard.** Overwork is another primary cause of fatigue. Many women are exhausted simply because they are trying to do too much and are running themselves into the ground trying to keep up with an unrealistic list of things to do. If you don't allow yourself time for relaxation and play, your body and psyche don't have the opportunity for rejuvenation. Even 30 minutes a day of time for yourself with no interruptions can go a long way toward restoring your energy.

- **Get plenty of sleep.** Most women are chronically sleep deprived. Go to bed early enough at night so that you are able to awaken naturally without the aid of an alarm. The earlier you go to bed before midnight, the better, because those are the hours that your body performs much of its restorative work. If you have trouble sleeping, drink a cup of relaxing herbal tea such as passion flower or chamomile, and take a warm bath with Epsom salts, which have relaxing properties. If you suffer from insomnia, see the suggestions in Chapter 15.

- **Resolve underlying emotional tension.** Inner tension in the form of unresolved emotions is often an underlying factor in fatigue, because anger, fear, grief, and anxiety cause emotional distress that drains emotional and physical energy. Make sure that you have a safe place to share your innermost feelings, either through journaling, with trusted friends, in women's groups, or through psychotherapy. Meditation and yoga are other ways of accessing your inner self, and they encourage a balance between body, mind, and spirit that allows for the free flow of energy and the building of vitality. Deep-relaxation and breathing exercises also promote a sense of peace and calm that helps to bring the body and psyche into harmonious balance. For suggestions for relaxation exercises, see Appendix II.

Essential Oils That Relieve Fatigue

Essential oils can either relax or energize you, depending on the oils you choose. Use relaxing scents such as lavender and clary sage in baths and massages to help you unwind after a stressful day and to promote a good night's sleep. Use stimulating essential oils such as basil, rosemary, and peppermint in cool baths or footbaths for a quick boost of energy.

Lavender has relaxing and restorative properties for the body and the psyche. It helps to relieve fatigue that is related to emotional tension and also eases muscle aches caused by physical exertion. Lavender has a floral herbaceous fragrance with balsamic undertones.

Clary sage is deeply relaxing and helps to relieve fatigue by calming an overly active mind and by enhancing adrenal function. It also helps to relax tense muscles and promotes restful sleep. Clary sage has a musty, deep, sweet scent.

Basil has an uplifting effect on the psyche and helps to dispel mental fatigue. It also enhances the function of the adrenal glands. Basil has a warm, sweet, spicy scent.

Rosemary is one of the most potent and balanced essential-oil stimulants for both the mind and the body. It enhances the functioning of the adrenal glands, helps to overcome fatigue, and also improves mental clarity. Rosemary has a strong, herbaceous fragrance with mint and camphor undertones.

Peppermint is energizing and invigorating and is excellent for relieving mental exhaustion and physical fatigue. It has a potent, minty scent, and because it is so strong, should be used only in small amounts (no more than three drops in a bath).

Energy-Restoring Bath

This bath combines the soothing qualities of lavender with the energizing effects of rosemary and peppermint for an uplifting, yet restorative bath.

7 drops lavender essential oil
3 drops rosemary essential oil
2 drops peppermint essential oil
1 cup sea salt
1 cup baking soda

Draw a bathtub of comfortably warm water. Combine sea salt and baking soda in a covered container and add essential oils. Shake well to combine, and add just before entering the tub. Soak for 15 minutes, and finish with a cool shower to energize your body and clear your mind.

Chapter 13

Transform Stress
and Anxiety

Midlife, and especially the menopausal years, is often associated with emotional upheaval in the form of mood swings, anxiety, depression, and insomnia. Because the mind and body are intricately intertwined, the physiological changes that occur during menopause have an effect on the psyche. Women's emotions are often blamed on shifting hormones, and while it's true that hormones play a role in your emotional state, it's important to realize that many life factors affect your emotional well-being, including relationships, family, health, and work. In addition, unresolved emotional issues from the past have a way of resurfacing at midlife. Emotional turmoil often has roots in both the psychological and the physiological, and healing into a place of balance takes place when both are attended to.

Your emotions, however uncomfortable they may be, provide a window into the deepest recesses of your being and can help you to get in touch with your true needs, desires, and dreams. It is important to not deny what you are feeling and to allow your emotions to lead you to a place of greater self-understanding. At the same time, you don't need to be debilitated by stress, anxiety, and depression.

Supporting your body with a healthful diet and herbs, getting enough exercise and rest, and building a strong emotional support system can help you to build the emotional and physical resilience that will help you to best cope with difficult times and feelings.

Reevaluating Stress

This may surprise you, but it's not possible, nor is it desirable, to live without stress. I once saw a t-shirt that said, "I can't relax—my stress is the only thing holding me together!" In a sense, that's true. Without some level of stress, we would be like blobs of Jell-O, unable to respond to the myriad experiences that life presents to us. Stress is simply the body's heightened physiological response to new situations and to the ever-changing conditions of life. Although we tend to think of stress only in negative terms—relationship difficulties, job pressures, family problems, and financial concerns— the stress response is also triggered by positive experiences, such as a new relationship, a promotion at work, and buying a home. While there is no doubt that positive stressors feel better than negative ones, positive stressors can lead to anxiety just as quickly as negative stressors. The key is learning to manage your life challenges so that you are not in *distress* and to prevent stress from taking a toll on your physical and emotional well-being. In this way, stress can lead to growth, self-confidence, and the ability to handle future stressors more easily.

People vary in their ability to handle stress, and what one woman finds devastating might not phase another at all. Events or situations don't inherently cause stress, but your interpretation and response to the event or situation does. Of course, there are difficult and tragic life events that cause most people to feel distress, but for the most part, the situations that cause stress in our lives are minor annoyances that we allow to consume us. Years ago, when I was studying to become a therapist, I learned a valuable technique that I still use to help me keep my life in perspective. Whenever I start to feel stressed about something, I stop and ask myself, "Is this going to matter 100 years from now?" The answer is always no. The truth is that most things aren't going to matter even next year, or next month, or tomorrow. It always helps me to put my life in perspective and to realize that there aren't too many things that are worth getting really worked up about.

Because the physiological changes that occur in response to stressful situations are largely unconscious, we may not be aware many times of what is happening until the tension erupts into a headache, backache, upset stomach, or racing heart. Stress, especially chronic, unresolved stress, takes a significant toll on your physical and emotional well-being—in fact, as many as 90 percent of all illnesses are stress-related. Common symptoms of stress include fatigue, anxiety, diarrhea, insomnia, headache, back pain, rapid heart rate, irritability, muscle tension, stomach upset, teeth grinding, loss of sexual interest, difficulty concentrating, and skin rashes. To add fuel to the fire, we all have our favorite ways that we've learned for dealing with stress, and they are often not healthful ways of coping. Alcohol, drugs, smoking, overeating, and watching too much television are just a few of the negative coping patterns that are prevalent in our society.

There are many positive, self-nurturing ways of managing stress. Creating a healthful lifestyle builds a strong foundation that enables you to meet the challenges of life with a minimum of wear and tear on your body and psyche. A nutrient-rich diet, regular exercise, and plenty of rest strengthens your physical resistance. Practicing calming and centering techniques such as deep relaxation and meditation and learning positive coping skills for areas of your life that are causing you stress helps to bolster your emotional well-being and gives you strength of spirit. Herbs can also be powerful allies for helping you to handle life stressors. Tonic herbs such as *ginseng* support the endocrine system, which plays a critical role in helping your body to more easily handle stress. Mild relaxing herbs such as *chamomile* and *lemon balm* can be used to promote a sense of calm, and stronger sedative and mood-elevating herbs such as *kava* can be taken on a short-term basis to relax the mind and body so that the deeper work of understanding emotional turmoil and learning new ways of coping can take place.

Anxiety: Stress Magnified

Anxiety is one of the most common symptoms of stress. All of us have experienced anxiety as a temporary reaction to a stressful situation. In such instances, a little anxiety is not a bad thing, because it sharpens our awareness and prepares us for the challenge that lies ahead. For many women, though, anxiety takes on a life of its own and becomes an underlying current of unrest that interferes with normal living. While some anxiety is normal, intense anxiety or anxiety that is chronic can cause physical and emotional health problems.

When we are anxious, we react physically as though danger is imminent. The autonomic nervous system is aroused, which speeds up heart rate and breathing, raises blood pressure, dumps stored sugars in the form of glucose into the bloodstream, and increases levels of hormones such as adrenaline and cortisol. Dubbed the "fight-or-flight response," this reaction is an automatic, unconscious life-saving instinct that evolved at the dawn of human history when, in order to survive, we needed the ability to either fight for our lives or flee from danger. The physiological changes that occur during the stress response supply the body with a sudden burst of energy and strength to deal with life-threatening danger. The problem is that our bodies don't distinguish between life-threatening danger (such as being chased by a wild animal or having a near collision on a freeway) and stressors such as job pressures and financial worries. Stressors that are well defined and short term are the easiest for your body to handle, because when the anxiety-provoking situation has passed, your body returns to a relaxed state of functioning. This is crucial, because your body needs this resting stage to come back into balance. Long-term, ill-defined stressors, such as the emotional stress that occurs with relationship, job, family, or money problems, can create a chronic state of anxiety that causes wear and tear on your body and psyche. Sooner or later, something breaks down.

Common symptoms of anxiety include heart palpitations, feelings of tightness in the chest, breathing difficulties, chest pain, headaches, muscle spasms, back pain, dizziness, digestive disturbances, insomnia, fear, and the nagging feeling that something bad is going to happen. Anxiety can range from mild nervousness to severe panic attacks and phobias, but it is always a signal that you are in distress and that you need to pay attention to your physical and emotional well-being. Tranquilizers are often prescribed for anxiety, and while they are effective, they are also extremely addictive and usually require increasingly larger doses over time to have a relaxing effect. They also have serious side effects such as mental confusion and grogginess and can cause rebound anxiety. In most cases, nondrug approaches such as relaxation training, meditation, and yoga are a better alternative. They are often more effective than drugs for mild to moderate anxiety and help you to learn skills for coping with stress. Because anxiety is often caused by a feeling of loss of control, learning to manage stress is empowering and freeing.

If you have a more severe manifestation of anxiety, such as phobias (where a specific object or activity elicits extreme fear) or panic attacks (severe, spontaneous attacks of anxiety that occur unpredictably, with feelings of doom and fears of dying or going crazy), seek professional help. A skilled therapist can help you to release yourself from the prison of disabling anxiety. Some health problems such as hypoglycemia, thyroid disorders, and hormonal imbalances associated with PMS and menopause can also cause feelings of anxiety. If your anxiety is severe or if you do not feel better after trying the suggestions in this chapter, consult your health-care practitioner.

Eating to Bolster Your Stress Resistance

A nutrient-rich diet is essential for building a strong foundation that will enable your body to cope with stressful situations. The surge of adrenaline that occurs as part of the physiological stress response increases the metabolism of protein, fats, and carbohydrates to produce the energy needed to deal with the crisis. Follow the guidelines in Chapter 26 for a health-enhancing diet. Take special care to avoid food stressors such as caffeine, alcohol, and refined carbohydrates.

Caffeine is a major contributor to feelings of anxiety. Even small amounts can cause restlessness, heart palpitations, headaches, insomnia, and overexcitability—all symptoms of anxiety. Make sure to cut out all sources of caffeine, including coffee, black tea, chocolate, cocoa, caffeinated soft drinks, coffee-flavored ice cream and candies, and over-the-counter medications that contain caffeine. Green tea also contains caffeine, and although it has healthful properties, if you are highly sensitive to caffeine you might be better off avoiding it. It's also best to not drink alcohol, because even though it is often used as a relaxant, it actually stresses your body through its effects on the endocrine and nervous systems and can intensify anxiety and irritability.

Overeating, particularly sweets and refined carbohydrates, is a favorite coping mechanism for many women. Food, especially sweets, can be soothing and sedating, but refined carbohydrates cause a rapid increase in blood-sugar levels that is quickly followed by a sharp drop. Swings in blood-sugar levels are hard on your body and can make you feel weak and fatigued, and if you are prone to hypoglycemia, can trigger feelings of anxiety. (See Chapter 17 for more information on hypoglycemia.) Instead, choose complex carbohydrates, which are found abundantly in whole grains, vegetables, legumes, fruits, seeds, and nuts. These healthful whole-food sugars help to stabilize blood-sugar levels and supply steady energy to your body and your brain. Eating plenty of fresh vegetables and fruits also ensures a rich supply of potassium, which is essential for strengthening the adrenal glands.

Other nutrients that are important for supporting adrenal health are vitamin C, pantothenic acid (vitamin B-5), vitamin B-6, magnesium, and zinc. Vitamin C is found in many fruits and vegetables, including cantaloupe, broccoli, red peppers, oranges, and strawberries. Rich sources of pantothenic acid include eggs, avocados, chicken, mushrooms, salmon, and yogurt. Lentils, tempeh, trout, tuna, avocados, and bananas are good sources of vitamin B-6. Zinc is found in pumpkin and sesame seeds, black beans, oysters, and mussels; magnesium-rich foods include almonds, corn, halibut, avocados, tofu, and peas. In addition to eating foods that supply these vital stress-combating nutrients, it's a good idea to take a high-potency vitamin and mineral supplement along with additional supplements if necessary to supply 2,000 milligrams of vitamin C, 50–100 milligrams of the B-complex vitamins, 400 milligrams of magnesium, and 30 milligrams of zinc.

Exercise Mindfully to Relieve Stress

Regular aerobic exercise is essential for relieving tension and anxiety and for building your resistance to stress. Exercise triggers the release of endorphins, your body's natural anxiety-relieving chemicals. Exer-

cise benefits you immediately by helping to burn off the stress-pro-
ducing hormones that are secreted by the adrenal glands, and engaging in regular exercise helps you to release tension on a daily basis
and prevents the accumulation of tension that can build into anxiety.

You can increase the stress-relieving benefits of exercise by
learning to exercise in a mindful way. Exercise alone reduces anxiety and strengthens your body against stress-related ills such as high
blood pressure and heart disease, and combining exercise with
meditation increases the psychological benefits. Adopting a practice
of engaging your mind while you are exercising enables you to
more quickly achieve a state of calm and relaxation. Oftentimes,
people who are highly stressed find that they take their problems
with them wherever they go, including while they are exercising.
Learning to exercise in a mindful way allows you to step away from
your stress and provides an opportunity to view the challenges you
are encountering in a more positive light.

To practice mindful exercise, choose a low-intensity aerobic
exercise such as walking (walking is perfect because it allows you
to move rhythmically and does not require concentration). Choose
a word or a phrase that you find soothing, such as a simple prayer,
a line from a poem, or a word. Some examples include "All is well,"
"I am safe," "Relax," or "Peace." As you walk, recite your chosen
word or phrase over and over, in rhythm with your steps. Repeating a word or phrase helps to quiet your mind and allows you to
concentrate on your body's movement and on your breathing.
When your mind wanders, gently bring your attention back to your
steps and begin again repeating your mindful phrase. The more you
practice, the easier mindful exercise becomes, until it becomes natural to leave your worries behind.

Two Yoga Poses for Relaxation

Yoga and tai chi are also wonderful forms of movement for practicing mindfulness and for enhancing relaxation. Both help to calm
and bring balance to the mind and the body and facilitate emotional and physical harmony through paying attention to the breath.
Two simple yoga postures that encourage a deep sense of peace
and relaxation are the head-to-knee pose and the child pose. Practice these poses daily, at any time of day that is convenient for you.

Head-to-Knee Pose

- Sit on the floor with your legs straight out in front of you. Bend your right leg and place your foot against the inside of your left thigh.
- Inhale, and reach up toward the ceiling to lengthen your spine.
- Exhale, and fold forward over your outstretched leg, clasping your calf, ankle, or foot (whichever you can comfortably hold).
- Concentrate on lengthening your spine and bringing your upper body toward your thigh. Keep your leg straight, and gently pull your body as close as you comfortably can to your leg.
- Hold the stretch for 30 seconds or longer, and return to the beginning position. Repeat on the opposite side.

Child Pose

- Kneel on the floor, sitting on your heels with your feet and knees close together.
- Bend forward from your waist and place your forehead on the floor.
- Place your arms beside your legs with your hands next to your feet and your palms facing upward.
- Rest, and breathe normally for one minute or as long as you desire.

Herbal Help for Stress and Anxiety

Herbs are not a cure for stress and anxiety, but they can be immensely helpful for both strengthening the endocrine system (which plays a key role in helping the body to adjust to stress) and also for calming emotional and physical tension. While it is helpful to use herbal sedatives for short-term relief of stress and anxiety, don't use herbs to cover up or suppress the root cause of these distressing emotions. Your psyche is speaking to you through your physical symptoms, and your symptoms will likely grow worse until you give them the attention they are asking for. A long-term approach to stress and anxiety is based on reestablishing balance through strengthening the endocrine and nervous systems. The adrenal glands, an integral part of the endocrine system, are key players in the body's response to stress. Chronic stress impairs adrenal function and can actually shrink the adrenals. Typical signs of adrenal exhaustion include feeling fatigued, stressed, and anxious.

Siberian ginseng and *American ginseng* are both excellent for strengthening the adrenal glands and for building resistance to stress and anxiety. One of these two herbs should definitely be part of your herbal program for managing stress. Both help to restore vitality, increase energy, and improve mental and physical performance. They also improve your body's response to stressful situations and help to moderate the detrimental effects of stress on your body. Gentle herbs such as *chamomile, linden flower, catnip,* or *lemon balm* may be sufficient for mild tension and can be used as daily beverage teas. Try these first if you are feeling generally stressed. Tonic herbs that help to restore balance to the nervous system include *St. John's wort* and *skullcap.* More powerful stress-relieving sedative herbs that are helpful during periods of intense anxiety include *kava* and *valerian.*

My friend Stephanie was debilitated by stress following a painful divorce that took place just as she was going through menopause. She found it increasingly difficult to function, and as her anxiety level increased so did her physical symptoms, which included tension headaches, backaches, and heart palpitations. She started taking American ginseng to strengthen her adrenal glands, along with kava to ease her anxiety. She also drank a blend of calming linden, chamomile, and motherwort three times a day as a replacement for coffee and black tea. Within a few days, her feelings of anxiety began to abate and she felt more able to cope with the life changes she was going through.

Adrenal Tonics

Siberian ginseng *(Eleutherococcus senticosus)* strengthens the immune, nervous, and endocrine systems, builds energy, and helps the body to adapt more easily to physical and emotional stressors. Take an extract standardized for eleutherosides, approximately 250 milligrams twice a day. Siberian ginseng is best used consistently for two months, with a two-week break before resuming the dosage. If you have high blood pressure, check with your doctor before using any type of ginseng.

American ginseng *(Panax quinquefolium)* has benefits similar to Siberian ginseng, but is a more potent tonic and is indicated for more severe, long-term stress. The potency of ginseng products varies greatly. Buy extracts standardized for ginsenosides, which are considered to be the active compounds, and follow the manufacturer's dosage recommendations. American ginseng is best used cyclically for two to three weeks at a time, followed by a two-week break. If you don't notice an appreciable difference within three cycles of using the herb, you may be using an inferior product and should try a different brand. If you have high blood pressure, consult with your doctor before taking ginseng. If you find that American ginseng makes you feel nervous or irritable or causes insomnia, decrease your dosage or try Siberian ginseng, which is milder.

Mild Stress-Relieving Herbs

Catnip *(Nepeta cataria)* is a mild, minty-tasting herb that helps to relieve tension and also eases nausea and digestive upsets. The essential oil in catnip that cats find so intoxicating has mild sedative properties for humans. Pour one cup of boiling water over one tablespoon of dried catnip. Cover, and steep for 15 minutes. Strain, sweeten if desired, and drink up to three to four cups a day.

Chamomile *(Matricaria recutita)* is one of the most popular herbal teas because of its delicate apple-like flavor. When made into a medicinal-strength infusion it also acts as a mild sedative. Chamomile can help to relieve tension headaches and digestive upsets related to stress. To make a medicinal infusion, pour one cup of boiling water over one tablespoon of dried chamomile. Cover, and steep for 15 minutes. Strain, sweeten if desired, and drink up to three to four cups a day.

Lemon balm *(Melissa officinalis)* is a mild, lemony-tasting herb with tension-relieving properties that has been used since the time of the ancient Greeks. The fragrant essential oil in lemon balm also has antispasmodic properties, which makes it helpful for digestive upsets. Pour one cup of boiling water over two to three teaspoons of dried lemon balm. Cover, and steep for 15 minutes. Strain, sweeten if desired, and drink three to four cups daily.

Linden *(Tilia vulgaris)*, also known as lime blossom, is a wonderful relaxing herb for nervous tension. It has a general relaxing effect on the circulatory system, which is helpful in cases of hypertension or migraine that are stress related. To make a delicious, slightly sweet and floral-tasting tea, pour one cup of boiling water over two teaspoons of dried linden blossoms. Cover, and steep for 15 minutes. Strain, sweeten if desired, and drink up to three cups daily.

More Potent Stress-Relieving Herbs

Motherwort *(Leonurus cardiaca)* has sedative properties and is a tonic for the cardiovascular system. It is especially helpful for nervous tension that manifests as heart palpitations and is a wonderful herbal ally for menopausal women. Motherwort has a bitter flavor. Pour one cup of boiling water over two teaspoons of dried motherwort, cover, and steep for 15 minutes. Strain, sweeten if desired, and drink three cups daily as needed, or take one-half teaspoon of liquid extract three times daily.

Skullcap *(Scutellaria laterifolia)* relieves nervous tension and is considered a tonic for the nervous system. It eases mood swings and stress-related headaches and is helpful for PMS. Skullcap has a slightly bitter flavor. Pour one cup of boiling water over two teaspoons of dried herb, cover, and steep for 15 minutes. Strain, sweeten if desired, and drink three cups daily, or take one-half teaspoon of liquid extract three times a day.

St. John's wort *(Hypericum perforatum)* is primarily known for its beneficial effects on depression, but it is also helpful for anxiety, which is often the flip side of depression. St. John's wort enhances the action of neurotransmitters in the brain that engender a positive, calm mood. Take 300 milligrams of an extract standardized to contain 0.3 percent hypericin, three times a day. The effect of hypericin is cumulative, not immediate, so you need to take the herb for at least six weeks to achieve beneficial results. If you are currently taking prescription antidepressants, consult with your health care practitioner before taking St. John's wort.

Herbs for Intense Stress and Anxiety

Kava *(Piper methysticum)* is a shrub native to the South Pacific, where the islanders make the root into a special drink that is used in ceremonies and celebrations because of its calming and euphoric properties. It has a natural tranquilizing and mood-elevating effect and relieves anxiety, tension, and insomnia. Kava is quick acting and is an excellent herb to use as a temporary measure to reestablish emotional balance when intense stress or anxiety are interfering with normal life. Kava has a very unpleasant taste when made into a tea. For best results, take an extract that provides 45 to 70 milligrams of kavalactones one to three times a day. Do not use kava with alcohol or prescription or herbal sedatives because it may dangerously intensify the sedative effects, and do not take kava if you have Parkinson's disease, because it may increase muscle twitching. Do not exceed the recommended dosage of kava, because although it is safe in recommended amounts, in large doses over an extended period of time it can cause a scaly skin condition.

Valerian *(Valeriana officinalis)* has been used for centuries in Ayurvedic and Chinese medicine to treat nervousness and insomnia and is a popular sedative in Europe. Research studies have found valerian to be as effective as the prescription drug Valium, but without the negative side effects. Valerian is a safe herbal sedative, but it should be reserved for those times when a strong tranquilizing effect is needed. For a small percentage of women, valerian can cause agitation instead of relaxation. If you've never used valerian, it's best to begin with a small dose to judge its effects on you and to then increase the dosage as needed. Valerian has a pungent, earthy odor and flavor. Take one-half teaspoon of extract or two capsules three times a day. If you wish to make a tea, pour one cup of boiling water over two teaspoons of the dried root, cover, and steep for 15 minutes. Strain, and drink up to three cups daily as needed. Do not exceed the recommended dosage, because large amounts can cause morning grogginess or headaches.

Gentle Calming Tea

1 tablespoon chamomile flowers
1 tablespoon linden flowers
1 tablespoon catnip
2 cups water

Pour boiling water over herbs, cover, and steep for 15 minutes. Strain, sweeten if desired, and drink up to 3 to 4 cups daily.

Herbal Sedative Tea

1 tablespoon valerian root
1 tablespoon skullcap
1 tablespoon linden flowers
2 cups water

Pour boiling water over herbs, cover, and steep for 15 minutes. Strain, sweeten if desired, and drink up to 3 cups daily for up to 2 weeks. This recipe can also be taken as a concentrated liquid extract. Buy one ounce each of valerian, skullcap, and linden extracts and combine in a dark-glass bottle. Shake well, and take one teaspoon 3 times a day with a small amount of warm water.

Aromatherapy for Easing Tension

Fragrant essential oils have powerful effects on the emotions and can help to relieve stress and anxiety when used in baths and massages, or even by placing a drop or two on a handkerchief and inhaling the fragrance. The following essential oils are especially helpful for easing emotional distress.

Bergamot has a sweet, spicy, citrusy fragrance. It has a refreshing and uplifting effect on the emotions and is helpful for both stress and anxiety. Bergamot contains a compound called bergapten that can cause skin photosensitivity, so use a bergapten-free oil.

Frankincense has a warm, rich, sweet balsamic fragrance and has been used as an incense since ancient times to promote a sense of peace and to soothe the spirit. It has sedative properties and slows and deepens the breathing, which helps to relieve stress and anxiety.

Lavender has a sweet, herbaceous, floral, and balsamic fragrance. It is balancing for the body and emotions and helps to relieve anxiety, nervous stress, and headaches or insomnia that are caused by tension.

Marjoram has a warm, herbaceous, slightly spicy fragrance. It has potent sedative properties, eases nervous tension and irritability, and is helpful for stress-related disorders such as muscle tension and headaches.

Rose has a sweet, floral, intensely rose fragrance. It has mild sedative and balancing effects on the psyche, is soothing and comforting, and promotes a feeling of well-being.

Sandalwood has a deep, rich, woodsy fragrance. It has mild sedative properties, engenders a sense of peaceful relaxation, and is helpful for relieving anxiety and all stress-related complaints. Burning sandalwood incense creates a peaceful atmosphere.

Ylang ylang has a very sweet, exotic floral fragrance and has a sedative and slightly euphoric effect on the emotions. It is helpful for both anxiety and nervous tension. A drop or two of ylang ylang is sufficient—beware of overdosing, because too much can cause headaches or nausea.

Body and Mind-Relaxing Bath

2 cups Epsom salts
1 cup baking soda
10 drops lavender essential oil
5 drops marjoram essential oil

Draw a tubful of warm water, and while the water is running add the Epsom salts and baking soda. After the tub has filled, mix the lavender and marjoram essential oils into the bathwater. Darken the room, light a candle, put on soothing music, and soak for 15–20 minutes. Imagine as the tub drains that all of your tension is draining away with the water.

Sandalwood-Floral Soothing Bath

5 drops sandalwood essential oil
5 drops rose essential oil
2 drops ylang-ylang essential oil

Add essential oils to a bathtub of warm water. Light a candle, play your favorite relaxing music, and sip a cup of hot linden-flower tea while you soak for 15–20 minutes.

Stress-Relieving Massage Oil

3 ounces almond oil
1 ounce jojoba oil
15 drops lavender essential oil
15 drops sandalwood essential oil
10 drops frankincense essential oil

Combine almond and jojoba oil with essential oils in a dark-glass bottle. Shake well, and store tightly capped in a cool, dark place.

Other Helpful Ways to Relieve Stress and Anxiety

Talk or Journal to Release Anxiety

Keeping fears, worries, and concerns bottled up inside is a primary contributor to emotional distress. One of the most helpful things you can do to relieve anxiety is to find someone you trust with whom you can share your feelings. If your stress or anxiety is great or long-standing, seek the help of a skilled therapist to help you to unravel the emotions that are causing you pain and to learn new ways of being comfortable in life. Keeping a journal can help immensely to break the patterns that lock you into stress and anxiety. Try writing in stream of consciousness, without censoring anything that you are feeling or thinking and without any thought of grammar, spelling, or writing well. Allow yourself the freedom to pour all of your thoughts and worries onto the paper. Journaling in this way helps to keep anxiety from building up. It may take a few sessions of writing, but once you have released all your fears and worries, you will naturally come to a place of calm and clarity that will allow solutions to emerge.

Practice Relaxation Exercises

Relaxation exercises are crucial for helping to relieve anxiety. Meditation, visualization, deep-breathing exercises, progressive relaxation, and prayer are just a few of the ways that you can calm your body and center your mind. Just taking the time to relax and be still lessens anxiety, because constantly running from one activity to the next activates the physiological stress response. When your mind and body are calm, it is impossible to feel stressed. Relaxation exercises are easy to learn and can be practiced anywhere. Choose a technique that appeals to you (see Appendix II for suggestions) and set aside at least ten minutes twice a day to practice. Conscious breathing exercises are especially helpful for relieving stress and anxiety, because deep relaxed breathing triggers a relaxation response that is the opposite of the stress response. Conscious breathing exercises take only a few minutes a day, and the more you practice them, the easier it will be to use your breath as a tool to help you relax as soon as you feel tension building.

Simplify Your Life

One of the primary stressors for many women is time, or rather, feeling the lack of it. It's important to set priorities and to accept that there is only so much you can accomplish in one day. If you constantly feel time pressured, take a thoughtful look at your life. You might find it helpful to write down how you spend your time, hour by hour, over the course of a week. The next step is to decide what is really important to you and to practice letting the rest go. Make sure that you are making time for yourself each day for self-nurturing, exercise, and relaxation. The more you give to yourself, the more you have to give to others. If your cup is empty, you don't have much to share. Ask other people for help, delegate responsibilities, and simplify your life.

Simplifying your life is a powerful way to create more time. Too many possessions create stress and drain your energy just by their sheer presence and the need to take care of them. If you are overwhelmed by the prospect of simplifying your life, take it one room at a time, or even one drawer or one closet at a time, and keep going until you have pared your possessions down to what is essential and to what brings beauty to your life and nourishes your spirit. Make your home a refuge that is peaceful and beautiful. Fill your sacred space with natural light, fresh air, plants, flowers, pleasing colors, soothing music, and wonderful fragrances. Everything in your surroundings affects you, so consciously create an environment that is deeply satisfying and relaxing.

Cultivate the Art of Conscious Living

Above all, what is most important is to practice being fully present *in this moment* in life and to realize that simply *being* is far more important than doing or having. It can be helpful to write down how you want to spend your time and your life energy. Imagine your ideal life as you would like it to be and journal about it or collage a visual image with pictures that you cut out from magazines. Writing down or creating a visual image of your deepest desires is a powerful tool for planting the seeds that can blossom into your ideal life.

Begin cultivating conscious moment-by-moment awareness so that tension does not have an opportunity to build. When you awaken in the morning, instead of immediately jumping out of bed, take a few minutes to begin your day in a peaceful way. Tune in to your body, and gently stretch your muscles. Become aware of your breathing, and spend a minute or two observing how your breath enters and leaves your body. Express your gratitude for another day of life, and visualize yourself moving through your day in a relaxed and conscious way. It's also helpful to get up 30 minutes earlier than usual to practice a few yoga postures or a centering meditation. Throughout the day, remind yourself every hour to check in with your breathing, and get up and move around and stretch to keep your energy flowing. In the late afternoon or early evening, take a brisk walk to let go of stress that might have accumulated during the day. Relax before bed in a warm bath, drink a cup of chamomile or linden tea, and take a few minutes to journal before sleeping to release any thoughts or feelings that might cause emotional tension.

Chapter 14

Overcome Depression Naturally

Everyone experiences grief and sadness at times, just as we experience happiness and joy. Moods come and go, and cycles of emotional ups and downs are a normal part of life. However, ongoing feelings of profound sadness that are accompanied by feelings of hopelessness, fatigue, difficulty in concentrating, disturbed sleep and eating habits, and a loss of pleasure in activities that you would normally find pleasurable are an indication of depression. The spectrum of depression ranges widely, from feeling low to serious contemplation of suicide. Depression can be caused by a number of factors, but it is usually the result of either a traumatic life event or an imbalance in brain chemistry.

The Causes of Depression

Situational depression is triggered by a stressful life event such as the death of a loved one, chronic illness, ongoing relationship problems, or job loss. Many women experience situational depression associated with midlife and the myriad changes that accompany this life transition, such as menopause, children leaving home, relationship changes, and the loss of youth. Obviously, deep sadness is a normal reaction to a major life loss or trauma. But after a period of grieving, it is also normal to accept the loss and to begin to enjoy life again. Physically based depression is usually caused by a biochemical disorder in the brain, and there is often a family history of depression, with the disorder occurring at midlife or later. Depression can also have physiological causes such as hypoglycemia, hypothyroidism, and hormonal imbalances triggered by PMS and menopause. If you are seriously or chronically depressed, see your doctor for a health evaluation to rule out physical disorders that may be causing the depression.

Antidepressants such as Prozac are commonly prescribed for treating depression, and while they are effective, they can also cause unpleasant side effects such as anxiety, agitation, and digestive disturbances. Antidepressants work by increasing levels of brain chemicals such as serotonin that have a natural mood-elevating and tranquilizing effect. Low levels of serotonin are associated with depression, anxiety, irritability, and the inability to concentrate, while high levels of serotonin are linked with feeling optimistic, calm, creative, patient, loving, and focused. Antidepressant drugs are not the only solution for balancing brain chemistry, however. Diet, exercise, nutritional supplements, and herbs are powerful tools for increasing levels of the natural mood-enhancing compounds that your body makes and for restoring emotional balance. Many doctors are too quick to write prescriptions for antidepressant drugs when lifestyle changes and natural remedies present a safer and healthier alternative. It is far better to avoid drugs, especially in cases of mild to moderate depression, and to use natural therapies combined with appropriate emotional work for healing the underlying psychological distress. *If you are suffering from depression that is severe enough to interfere with your normal daily functioning or if you have thoughts of suicide, consult a mental-health-care professional for guidance.*

The Midlife Blues

Many women find that the perimenopausal and menopausal years bring profound and disturbing emotions to the surface. This is a time of great change, and fluctuating hormones add to the physiological and psychological transformation. It is extremely important during this time not to suppress your feelings, but to honor them. There is often wisdom and greater self-understanding lying beneath the surface of depression. Many women have spent years denying the truth about who they are and what they feel, and depression may be the self crying out for acknowledgment. Midlife is a time for reflecting on what your life has been thus far, and you may find that you grieve paths not taken, opportunities missed, and the loss of youth. Giving yourself the time to fully explore your feelings will help you to free yourself from regrets and to make decisions as to how you want to live in the present.

Meditation and other practices that are centering can be especially helpful for finding and nourishing a stable emotional core and cultivating a sense of inner peace. We aren't taught how to be peaceful and balanced in our culture. Instead, we are led to believe that we should be ecstatically happy all of the time and that if we are not, then we need to do something about it as quickly as possible. Focusing on cultivating peace of mind and serenity is a much healthier goal than striving for the emotional and transient high of happiness. From a place of emotional balance, happiness and joy are a delight to experience, but there is not a sense of something lacking if you are not feeling ecstatically happy twenty-four hours a day.

Nutritional Help for Depression

What you eat has a powerful effect on your mood—in fact, psychological disturbances are one of the first symptoms of nutrient deficiencies. Your brain requires an adequate and steady supply of nutrients and quickly shows signs of stress when your diet is inadequate. Nerve cells in the brain communicate through chemicals called neurotransmitters, which are dependent upon specific nutrients in the blood. Antidepressants work by increasing levels of neurotransmitters, but you can also increase these mood-elevating substances with foods and nutritional supplements. For a strong nutritional foundation that supplies your brain with the building blocks it needs for emotional well-being, eat a nutrient-dense, whole-foods diet. Follow the suggestions in Chapter 26, and pay special attention to maintaining stable blood-sugar levels, because the brain and nervous system are highly sensitive to blood-sugar fluctuations. Avoid sugar, caffeine, and alcohol, and eat small meals several times a day centered around high-complex carbohydrates, lean proteins, and healthful fats to ensure a steady supply of nutrients that help to keep blood-sugar levels balanced. Protein-rich foods such as chicken, turkey, fish, tofu, eggs, lentils, almonds, and yogurt are particularly important for overcoming depression because they are made up of amino acids, which are the building blocks for mood-elevating neurotransmitters. Eat a small serving of protein-rich food at each meal (approximately 8–10 ounces per day total) and snack on a few almonds, walnuts, or other raw nuts and seeds a couple of times a day.

Essential fatty acids are another important nutrient for alleviating depression because they play a critical role in maintaining healthy cell membranes, which are involved in the synthesis and transmission of neurotransmitters. Depression is associated with low levels of essential fatty acids, particularly gamma linolenic acid (GLA) and omega-3 fatty acids. GLA is found in capsules of evening primrose, black currant, and borage oil. Take enough capsules to equal between 120 and 240 milligrams of GLA daily. Omega-3 fatty acids are found in cold-water fish (salmon, mackerel, sardines), flaxseeds, and walnuts. Take one tablespoon of flaxseed oil daily, and eat omega-3 rich fish two or three times a week.

Since low levels of many nutrients are associated with depression, it's helpful to take a high-potency vitamin and mineral supplement that contains 50 to 100 milligrams of the B-complex vitamins. Vitamin B-12 is especially important for alleviating depression. Because it is not easily assimilated, use sublingual tablets of B-12, which are dissolved under the tongue and absorbed directly into the bloodstream. Take one milligram every other day.

Banish Depression with Exercise

Exercise is one of the most powerful tools you have available for banishing depression. Regular daily exercise has been proven to be as effective as antidepressant drugs for relieving mild to moderate depression, and in contrast to pharmaceutical drugs, has only beneficial health-enhancing side effects. Aerobic exercise stimulates the release of endorphins, the body's natural mood-elevating compounds. It also offers a healthy outlet for burning off feelings of anger and frustration and provides a sense of empowerment for coping with the challenges that life presents. The minimum amount of exercise that is effective for relieving depression is approximately 30 minutes of activity five days a week.

Early morning exercise seems to be most helpful for establishing a balanced and positive mood for the day, but exercise is beneficial at any time. Try taking a brisk walk the next time you feel low; it is an immediate and effective way to quickly shift your mood.

Herbal Help for Depression

An herbal strategy for relieving depression focuses not only on easing the depression, but also includes herbs that help to restore balance to the endocrine and nervous systems. Because depression is often accompanied by lack of energy and insomnia, it is helpful to take energizing herbs such as *ginseng* in the morning and herbs that encourage restful sleep such as *passionflower* and *skullcap* at night. For more suggestions on relieving fatigue and insomnia, see Chapters 12 and 15. The following are the most helpful herbs for treating depression:

St. John's wort *(Hypericum perforatum)* has become extremely popular in the past few years for easing depression. It has been used for centuries to treat depression and has been proven to be as effective as pharmaceutical antidepressants but without the negative side effects such as anxiety, insomnia, fatigue, and nausea. St. John's wort also helps to relieve insomnia, which often accompanies depression. For the most consistent results, take an extract of St. John's wort standardized to contain 0.3 percent hypericin, which is recognized as the active ingredient. Take 300 milligrams three times per day. It usually takes one or two months of regular use to produce the desired mood-elevating effect, but the same is true for prescription antidepressants. If you are currently taking antidepressant medication, consult with your doctor before taking St. John's wort because the herb may intensify the effects of the drug. Work with your doctor to gradually make the transition to St. John's wort by gradually tapering off your antidepressant medication. Avoid intense sun exposure while taking St. John's wort, because although it is unlikely, the herb may cause skin photosensitivity.

Ginkgo *(Ginkgo biloba)* is best known for improving memory, but it can also improve mood because depression in people over 50 can be caused by decreased blood flow to the brain. Older people are also more susceptible to depression because the number of serotonin receptor sites on brain cells decreases with age. Ginkgo increases blood flow to the brain by dilating the arteries and improving circulation, and preliminary studies show that it increases the number of serotonin receptor sites. Take 120 to 240 milligrams daily of an extract standardized for 24 percent ginkgo flavone glycosides.

Siberian ginseng *(Eleutherococcus senticosus)* strengthens the nervous and endocrine systems and restores healthy adrenal function. The adrenal glands play a critical role in the body's ability to adapt to physical and emotional stressors. Emotional and physical stress is a primary cause of adrenal fatigue, and weak adrenal function is clearly associated with depression. Take a standardized extract of Siberian ginseng, approximately 250 milligrams twice daily. Take Siberian ginseng consistently for two months, with a two-week break before resuming the dosage. Avoid taking near bedtime, because ginseng can be stimulating.

In cases of serious depression, standardized extracts are the most certain way of obtaining the recommended amounts of an herb's active ingredients. If you suffer from mild depression and want to make your own antidepressant formula, try the following recipe. If you do not obtain noticeable results within six weeks, switch to standardized extracts.

Mood-Elevating Formula

---

1 ounce St. John's wort extract
1 ounce Siberian ginseng extract
1/4 ounce licorice root extract
1/4 ounce ginger root extract

Combine the herbal extracts and store in a dark-glass bottle. Take 1/2 teaspoon 3 times a day in a small amount of warm water.

Lift Your Spirits with Aromatherapy

Essential oils have a direct influence on the limbic portion of the brain, which is the center of the brain responsible for emotions and memory. That's why smells evoke such immediate and powerful memories and feelings. Essential oils have a subtle and profound effect on the psyche and can be incorporated into your daily life in many ways to uplift your spirits and balance your emotions. Just the act of using essential oils is healing, because the more things you you do to nurture yourself, the better you will feel.

The following essential oils are especially helpful for relieving depression and can be used daily in baths and massage oils.

Bergamot has a fresh, spicy, citrusy fragrance and has an uplifting effect on the psyche. Bergamot contains bergapten, which can cause skin photosensitivity. Buy bergapten-free essential oil.

Lavender has a sweet, herbaceous, floral fragrance and is balancing for the nervous system. It acts as a restorative tonic and has antidepressant properties.

Rose has a sweet, floral, intensely rose fragrance. It promotes a feeling of well-being, eases sorrow and psychological pain, and opens the heart to feelings of love.

Sandalwood has a rich, woody, sweet fragrance. It has antidepressant effects and is also calming and harmonizing.

Mood Uplifting Massage Oil

---

3 ounces almond oil
1 ounce jojoba oil
20 drops lavender essential oil
10 drops rose essential oil
10 drops bergamot essential oil

Combine almond and jojoba oils with essential oils in a dark-glass bottle. Store in a cool, dark place, and shake well before using.

Fragrant Baths to Relieve Depression

Choose one of the following combinations of essential oils and add to a bathtub of warm water. Soak for 15 to 20 minutes. If you are feeling tense, add 2 cups of Epsom salts to the bath, which are rich in magnesium, a tension-relieving mineral.

*   **Rose-Bergamot Bath:** *5 drops rose, 5 drops bergamot*
    Sandalwood-Lavender Bath: *10 drops lavender,*
        5 drops sandalwood
    Lavender-Bergamot Bath: *10 drops lavender,*
        5 drops bergamot

Uncovering the Message Beneath Depression

While it is important to take positive steps to relieve depression, it is equally important to pay attention to the messages that your psyche is trying to give you. If you are feeling down, take time for reflection. What is calling for your attention? Depression is usually accompanied by a feeling of wanting to withdraw, which might be just exactly what you need to do for a day or two. Take some time out, and allow yourself to rest, to go inward, and to allow the feelings that are buried to surface. Depression is sometimes referred to as anger turned inward. Ask yourself what you might be angry or frustrated about, and try journaling or talking with a trusted friend about your feelings. Often, when you allow the full expression of your feelings, the depression will lift naturally. If you are severely depressed or if your depression continues for more than a couple of weeks, seek help. Chronic depression needs to be evaluated by a mental-health practitioner.

Depression is often related to low-self esteem and negative, self-defeating thoughts. If you are troubled by chronic or recurrent bouts of depression, consider cognitive therapy, which has been shown to be as beneficial as antidepressant drugs in treating mild to moderate depression. In cognitive therapy, you learn to recognize and dispute the unconscious negative thoughts that permeate your thinking and to replace them with more realistic and self-affirming thoughts. An excellent self-help book is *Feeling Good,* by David Burns, M.D.

Finally, do as much as you can to nurture yourself when you are feeling down. Use relaxation practices such as meditation, deep breathing, and visualization. See the suggestions in Appendix II for a variety of relaxation techniques. Massage and other forms of body-work can also be a helpful tool for releasing deep emotions, and touch is wonderfully healing for the body and the spirit. Spend time in nature, watch a favorite film, read something inspiring, listen to uplifting music. When you have allowed yourself the time to feel all of your feelings, begin to take positive steps to return to living fully.

Chapter 15

Sleep Well
Every Night

Most women need about seven or eight hours of sleep each night to wake up feeling refreshed. But many factors interfere with a good night's rest, including stress, tension, anxiety, and depression. Insomnia, or difficulty falling or staying asleep, can also be caused by stimulants such as caffeine and environmental factors such as loud noises and bright lights. The hormonal fluctuations that occur with PMS and menopause are also prime contributors to sleep difficulties. Over-the-counter and prescription sedatives are the most common treatments for insomnia, but although they knock you out they don't provide restful sleep and often cause grogginess and fatigue the next day. In addition, prescription sedatives are powerfully addictive, and even over-the-counter sedatives can be habit forming. There are many simple, natural, and effective remedies for relieving insomnia, from diet and lifestyle changes to herbs and essential oils that will help you to safely get a restful, healing night's sleep.

Adjusting Your Diet for a Good Night's Sleep

Eliminating all sources of caffeine is essential for preventing and relieving insomnia. Some women are especially sensitive to the stimulating effects of caffeine, and even one cup of coffee in the morning can interfere with sleep patterns that night. Be scrupulous about avoiding coffee, black tea, colas and other caffeinated soft drinks, chocolate, cocoa, and coffee-flavored foods such as ice cream, yogurt, and candies. Even the trace of caffeine found in decaffeinated coffee and tea can be enough to keep you awake at night. Many over-the-counter drugs contain ingredients that can cause insomnia; for example, some pain relievers and medications to relieve PMS contain caffeine, and some decongestants contain pseudoephedrine, a powerful stimulant.

Alcohol also causes sleep problems, because it stimulates the release of adrenaline and inhibits the transport of the amino acid tryptophan into the brain. Tryptophan is necessary for the production of serotonin, a compound that enhances sleep. A mug of warm milk is a time-honored bedtime remedy that can help induce sleep because it contains tryptophan. If you prefer to avoid dairy products, drink soy milk or almond milk instead. Sweeten your beverage of choice with a bit of honey or maple syrup and vanilla and add a pinch of freshly grated nutmeg, an Ayurvedic remedy for insomnia. Milk and almond milk (and calcium-fortified soy milk) are also rich in calcium, which helps to relax the nervous system and the muscles. For this reason, many women find that taking supplements of calcium and magnesium at bedtime ensures restful sleep. Take 800 to 1,200 milligrams of calcium and 400 to 600 milligrams of magnesium about an hour before bed.

Maintaining stable blood-sugar levels during the night is important, because nighttime drops in blood sugar can cause awakening. Eating too many refined carbohydrates and sweets can cause blood-sugar instability. If nighttime hypoglycemia is a problem, have a snack such as a small bowl of whole-grain cereal or a piece of toast about 30 minutes before bedtime. In addition to helping to maintain stable blood-sugar levels, high-complex carbohydrates may also stimulate the production of the brain's natural sedative neurotransmitters.

Exercise to Prevent Insomnia

Regular daily aerobic exercise such as a 30-minute brisk walk helps to relieve stress and promotes physical relaxation, but avoid strenuous exercise late in the day because it can be overstimulating. A gentle after-dinner walk is fine and can even help to ensure a restful night's sleep.

Yoga and tai chi are excellent for relieving the physical and emotional tension that can interfere with sleep. Deep-breathing and relaxation exercises help the body and mind to unwind and create a state of peaceful balance that enhances sleep. Practice relaxation and deep-breathing exercises just before bed, or even while you are in bed preparing for sleep. Try the following deeply relaxing yoga pose:

THE SPONGE

- Lie flat on your back with your legs a comfortable distance apart. Rest your arms next to your body with your palms facing upward.

- Close your eyes, and scan your body for any areas of tension. Consciously relax those areas.

- Use your breath to help you relax. With each inhalation, imagine that you are breathing in relaxation. With each exhalation, imagine that you are breathing out tension.

- Remain in this pose for at least five minutes or for as long as you choose to.

Anna suffered from chronic insomnia for years and relied on over-the-counter sleep aids that left her feeling drowsy and irritable. She has found that drinking a cup of warm soy milk with nutmeg and practicing a deep-breathing and relaxation exercise before going to bed enables her to sleep well almost every night. On the occasions when she still has difficulty sleeping, she takes *valerian,* an herbal sedative, and if she feels particularly tense, she makes sure to soak in a relaxing aromatherapy bath before bed.

Herbal Help for Insomnia

Even if you don't suffer from insomnia, you might want to cultivate the habit of drinking a cup of relaxing herbal tea before bed. For mild insomnia, it might be all you need to ensure a good night's rest. Teas made from *lemon balm* and *passionflower* have been used as sleep aids for centuries. More difficult cases of insomnia may call for more powerful sedative herbs such as *valerian, hops,* and *kava*. These potent sedative herbs are safe, but should not be relied upon night after night for helping you to sleep. When your life and your body are in balance and your mind is calm and centered, you will naturally sleep in a peaceful, sound manner. Sedative herbs can be useful to help restore normal sleep patterns, but don't use them to cover up the problems that are causing the sleep disturbance.

St. John's wort can be helpful for relieving chronic insomnia that is caused by anxiety or depression. St. John's wort does not provide immediate relief—it usually takes a couple of months of consistent use to begin to feel the effects. If you want to try St. John's wort, take an extract standardized to contain 0.3 percent hypericin, 300 milligrams three times a day. The following herbs are some of the most helpful for treating insomnia.

Mild Sleep-Enhancing Herbs

California poppy *(Eschscholzia california)* is a member of the opium poppy family. It contains natural chemicals that have a sedative effect similar to that of codeine, but it is much milder and not addictive. It is effective for nervous tension and anxiety that interfere with sleep. Pour one cup of boiling water over two teaspoons of dried herb, cover, and steep for 15 minutes. Strain, and sweeten if desired.

Lemon balm *(Melissa officinalis)* has been used for centuries as a mild tranquilizer, and in Germany it is a popular ingredient in herbal sedatives for insomnia. It has a light, lemony flavor and makes a mild sedative tea. Pour one cup of boiling water over two teaspoons of dried lemon balm. Cover, and steep for 15 minutes. Strain, and sweeten if desired.

Passionflower *(Passiflora incarnata)* has been used for centuries by Native Americans and Europeans as a sleep aid and is included in many sleep preparations in Britain and Germany. It has mild tranquilizing and sedative properties and promotes restful sleep. To make a pleasant-tasting tea, pour one cup of water over two teaspoons of dried herb, cover, and steep for 15 minutes. Strain, and sweeten if desired.

More Powerful Sedative Herbs

Hops *(Humulus lupulus)* is a potent sedative that has a relaxing effect on the central nervous system (it's one of the primary ingredients used in making beer). Hops is a good alternative for women who find that valerian causes agitation (see "Valerian," below). However, if you are prone to depression, avoid using hops because it is a central nervous-system depressant. It can be difficult to find good-quality dried hops because the active ingredients break down quickly. Buy dried hops that are strongly aromatic and have a rich, golden-green color. Extracts tend to preserve more of the active ingredients. To make a tea, pour one cup of boiling water over one to two teaspoons of dried hops. Cover, and steep for 15 minutes. Strain, and sweeten if desired. Hops has a pleasantly bitter, rich flavor. As an alternative, take one-half teaspoon of liquid extract in a small amount of warm water.

Kava *(Piper methysticum)* has a natural tranquilizing effect and is especially helpful for insomnia that is caused by anxiety. It contains compounds called kavalactones that are central nervous-system depressants and muscle relaxants. In small doses, kava acts to elevate mood, and in larger doses it acts as a sedative. Kava has a bitter, unpleasant flavor and is best used as an extract. Take one-half teaspoon of liquid extract or two capsules with warm water one hour before retiring. If you wish to take a standardized extract of kava, take enough capsules to provide 180 to 210 milligrams of kavalactones one hour before bed (approximately two to three capsules of an extract standardized for 60 to 75 milligrams of kavalactones per capsule).

Valerian *(Valeriana officinalis)* has been used for hundreds of years in China, India, and Europe to treat insomnia and is excellent as a nonaddictive sleep aid. It calms the nervous system and helps to quickly induce sleep. For a small percentage of women, valerian causes agitation instead of relaxation. If you've never used valerian before it's best to begin with a small dose and then to increase the amount if you have positive results. If you find it to be stimulating, try hops or kava instead. Because valerian has a very pungent odor and flavor, most women find it easier to take it as an extract or in capsules. To use valerian as a sedative for sleep, you need to use a larger amount than if you are using it to simply relieve anxiety. Take one to two teaspoons of valerian extract or two to three capsules with a small amount of warm water 30 minutes before bed. If necessary, repeat the dose after 30 minutes.

Gentle Sleep Tea

1 teaspoon California poppy
1 teaspoon passionflower
1 teaspoon lemon balm
1 cup water

Pour one cup of boiling water over herbs. Cover, and steep for 15 minutes. Strain, sweeten if desired, and drink 30 minutes before bedtime.

Insomnia-Relief Formula

1 ounce valerian root extract
1/2 ounce hops extract
1/2 ounce passionflower extract

Combine herbal extracts in a dark-glass bottle. Store in a cool, dark place and shake well before using. Take one teaspoon 30 minutes before bedtime with a small amount of warm water, and repeat the dose if needed. If you are sensitive to valerian, omit it and double the amount of hops extract.

Herbal Sleep Pillow

Small pillows stuffed with dried herbs have been used for centuries in Europe to promote restful sleep. Hops is a potent sedative, and lavender, chamomile, and rose petals all have relaxing, soothing properties.

1/8 cup dried hops
1/8 cup dried lavender
1/8 cup dried chamomile
1/8 cup dried rose petals
5 drops lavender or rose essential oil
2 pieces fabric, each 7 inches square

Mix the herbs together and sprinkle with the essential oil. Make a small pillowcase by sewing the right sides of the fabric together, leaving a 3-inch opening in the center of one side seam. Turn the pillowcase right side out. Fill the pillow with the dried herbs, making it fairly flat, and sew the opening closed. Slip the herbal sleep pillow underneath your bed pillow.

Aromatherapy for Sleep Enhancement

Essential oils act quickly on the brain and nervous system to induce relaxation and also help to ease muscle tension that can interfere with sleep. Taking a warm aromatherapy bath at night is a wonderful way to prepare for a restful night's sleep. Sip a cup of relaxing herbal tea, dim the lights, and soak for 15 to 20 minutes. Be sure to slip right into bed after your bath—don't distract yourself with other tasks that might stimulate your nervous system. The following essential oils are especially helpful for relieving insomnia.

Chamomile has a herbaceous, sweet and slightly tart fragrance that helps to relieve insomnia caused by nervous tension. Roman chamomile *(Anthemis nobilis)* tends to have a sweeter fragrance than German chamomile *(Matricaria recutita).*

Clary sage has potent sedative effects on the nervous system and has a slightly euphoric effect that is helpful for relieving insomnia. It also has muscle-relaxing properties. Clary sage has a warm, sweet, musty scent.

Lavender has soothing, sedating, and balancing effects on the mind and body. It has a floral, herbaceous fragrance with sweet or balsamic undertones.

Marjoram eases muscular and nervous tension and has relaxing and sedative effects. It has a sweet, spicy herbaceous fragrance.

Sweet-Dreams Bath

5 drops lavender essential oil

3 drops marjoram essential oil

3 drops clary sage essential oil

2 cups Epsom salts

1 cup baking soda

Draw a bathtub of warm (but not too hot) water, adding the Epsom salts and baking soda while the water is running. Add the essential oils to the bath just before entering the tub, mixing the oils into the water with your hand. Sip a cup of relaxing passionflower or lemon balm tea, and soak for 15–20 minutes. Immediately slip into bed after toweling dry.

Lifestyle Suggestions for Overcoming Insomnia

To help to ensure peaceful sleep, consciously begin slowing down a couple of hours before going to bed. Avoid working or engaging in any mentally or physically stressful activities in the evening, and spend the evening instead reading a relaxing book or watching a film, listening to peaceful music, or taking a soothing bath. Let go of the accumulated concerns of the day through journaling or relaxation exercises. Establish a regular bedtime, and try to stick to it even on the weekends. Your body responds best to a regular schedule, and you can train yourself to become sleepy at a specific time each evening. Go to bed early, before 10:00 P.M., to take advantage of your body's natural circadian rhythm of getting drowsy at dark and awakening at dawn.

Make sure your bedroom is a quiet, peaceful haven for sleep. Even a dim light can disturb sleep, so make your bedroom as dark as possible. Invest in room-darkening shades if necessary to block out external light. If noise is a problem, you can try soft earplugs, but they can be uncomfortable to wear. A better solution is an environmental sound machine that creates soothing background "white noise," such as gentle ocean waves, that blocks out all disturbing noise. You'll sleep better with plenty of fresh air, so keep your windows open at least a few inches, even in the winter.

Disrupted sleep is often caused by an unhealthful bedroom environment. Most mattresses, pillows, and bed linens are saturated with chemicals that release toxins such as formaldehyde into the air for years, causing symptoms such as headaches, nausea, fatigue, throat and eye irritation, and insomnia. When you consider that you spend approximately one-third of your life in bed, it makes sense to make your bedroom as healthful and comfortable as possible. Buy natural cotton sheets that have not been treated with chemicals (avoid any that are labeled "no-iron" or "easy care"). Cotton-flannel sheets are also a good option, especially for cooler months, and are naturally wrinkle-free. Layer your bed with cotton or wool blankets and down comforters, and instead of synthetic foam mattresses and pillows, choose cotton- or wool-filled mattresses and cotton-, down-, or wool-filled pillows. (Check the resource section for information on where to buy natural bedding.) For the most refreshing sleep, avoid mattresses that are too soft or too hard. A firm mattress that provides comfortable support for your back is best.

Avoid any activity in bed except sleep and sex. Don't read in bed, watch television, talk on the phone, or work. If you are unable to sleep, don't lie there and try to make yourself go to sleep or worry about it. Get up and do something relaxing, but not something that is too interesting—reading a boring book can be especially good for inducing sleep. As soon as you feel sleepy, go back to bed. If you again find that you can't sleep, repeat the process, and do it as many times as you need to until you finally fall asleep. It may take a couple of weeks, but this is a good way to train yourself to go to sleep, because you aren't fueling your anxiety about not being able to sleep. Avoid napping during the day, especially in the late afternoon, because it can interfere with nighttime sleep patterns.

In most cases, these simple suggestions will help you to overcome insomnia. If you are still having trouble sleeping after a month, you might want to try using supplements of melatonin. Melatonin is a hormone secreted by the pineal gland that regulates the body's circadian rhythm, your natural biological clock that governs cycles of waking and sleeping. The production of melatonin naturally increases at night, which causes you to become sleepy, and drops off in the morning as you get ready to awaken. Many problems with insomnia are related to a deficiency of melatonin, or melatonin being produced at the wrong time. Melatonin can help to reset your body's biological time clock. You can boost your body's natural production of melatonin by darkening your bedroom at night, eating a complex carbohydrate snack before bed, avoiding stimulants such as coffee, alcohol, and tobacco, and going for an early-morning walk each day to help to reset your body's natural circadian rhythm.

Melatonin appears to be safe, but it should be used only after other natural remedies have been tried because it can cause side effects such as fatigue, grogginess, headaches, and depression, although these effects are usually associated with taking too much of the hormone. Melatonin is most helpful for treating insomnia related to jet lag or temporary sleep disturbances. For this purpose, take from 0.5 to 3 milligrams a couple of hours before bed for several days. Consult your doctor before using melatonin if you suffer from any type of physical illness or depression.

Chapter 16

Keep Your Memory Sharp

Have you had the experience of walking into a room, only to forget what you were intending to do there? Or do you find yourself looking absently into the refrigerator, wondering what in the world you were looking for? Have you suddenly forgotten a close friend's name when you needed to introduce her to someone? Many women fear that these signs—along with misplacing keys and glasses, or forgetting well-known phone numbers and address-es—are signposts of mental deterioration on the road to Alzheimer's disease. It is true that senility, including Alzheimer's, is common among the elder-ly (approximately 10 percent of women over the age of 60 and 25 percent of women over the age of 85 suffer from some degree of Alzheimer's), and researchers are still not certain of the causes. How-ever, memory loss for most women is not caused by Alzheimer's, but instead by lifestyle factors. There are a number of things you can do to preserve your cognitive abilities—including eating well and exercising to nourish healthy brain function, taking herbs to support your brain and nervous system, and using meditation, relaxation, and intellectual stimulation to keep your mental functioning sharp.

Mental-Pause: How Menopause Affects Your Brain

Many women notice changes in their cognitive functioning as they enter the menopausal years, describing symptoms such as forgetfulness and poor concentration. One of the most humorous was a woman who told me that she felt as though she were going through "mental-pause." Memory impairment and difficulties in concentrating are common symptoms of menopause and are associated with fluctuating hormone levels, particularly a decrease in estrogen. The part of the brain connected with learning and memory (the hippocampus) contains estrogen receptors and is affected by circulating levels of estrogen. When estrogen levels decline, memory also takes a nosedive. The memory loss and other symptoms of cognitive decline that are linked to hormonal changes generally resolve as the body and brain adjust to lower levels of hormones. You can support this adjustment by eating well and taking herbs that help to balance your hormones (see the suggestions in Chapter 10). In addition, many women find it helpful to acknowledge that they need some "time out" from schedules and commitments and the linear way of thinking that our culture values so highly. Menopause is a time of great transition, and your difficulties in concentrating and memory loss may be a signal that you need to take more time to go inward, to seek your inner wisdom, and to discover how you wish to proceed with the second half of your life. At the same time, there are many simple things you can do to support optimal brain health and to lessen the possibility that you will ever have to endure a decline in mental functioning.

Mental decline is far from inevitable—recent studies have shown that with proper mental stimulation, we continue to grow new brain cells in the hippocampus even in our seventies. As with most degenerative diseases, mental deterioration is primarily caused by an unhealthful diet and lifestyle. Most of the decrease in mental functioning that women experience with aging is not the result of growing older, but instead is caused by atherosclerosis, which narrows the arteries that lead to the brain and cuts down on the brain's supply of oxygen and nutrients. Through diet, exercise, and herbs, you can improve circulation to your brain and greatly enhance your mental functioning.

Nutrition for Optimal Brain Function

Your brain needs an optimal supply of virtually every known nutrient to function properly. Nutrients help to build neurotransmitters, which are the way that nerve cells pass information to one another. Your memory function is directly related to how efficiently your nerve cells transmit information. Follow the guidelines for a health-enhancing diet in Chapter 26 to provide your body and your brain with a nutrient-rich diet. A common cause of mental fatigue and poor concentration is unstable blood-sugar levels, such as occurs with hypoglycemia. Your brain depends on a steady supply of glucose to function well, and if glucose levels fall too low, mental confusion, memory impairment, and mood swings are likely to result. Eat small meals every two to three hours to maintain a stable supply of nutrients in your bloodstream. For more information on hypoglycemia, refer to Chapter 17.

Pay special attention to avoiding the harmful fats—polyunsaturated oils, hydrogenated oils, and saturated fats—that are a primary cause of atherosclerosis (narrowing and hardening of the arteries). At the same time, make sure to eat sufficient amounts of healthful fats, especially omega-3 essential fatty acids, which are associated with optimal brain function. Omega-3 fatty acids help to maintain the flexibility of cell membranes, which allows nutrients to be more readily absorbed into brain and nerve cells and enhances the transmission of information between cells. Eat cold-water fish such as salmon, mackerel, sardines, and tuna three times a week, and take one tablespoon of flaxseed oil daily. Make sure that your cholesterol and triglyceride levels stay within healthy ranges, and follow the suggestions in Chapters 22 and 23 if you have high cholesterol levels or atherosclerosis. Also make sure to keep your blood pressure below 140/90, because elevated blood pressure injures the small blood vessels in the brain and is a primary cause of mental deterioration. High blood pressure also causes the small strokes that are a major factor in impaired mental function. If you have high blood pressure, follow the suggestions in Chapter 24.

Your brain uses more oxygen than any other organ in your body, which means that it is also exposed to a greater number of free radicals than any other organ. Free-radical damage is more than likely a primary factor in mental deterioration, including Alzheimer's disease. Eating lots of fresh vegetables and fruits keeps your bloodstream well supplied with antioxidants, which help to guard against free-radical damage, as well as numerous other phytochemicals that protect your brain cells. In addition, taking a variety of antioxidant supplements such as vitamin C, vitamin E, beta-carotene and other carotenes, CoQ-10, zinc, and selenium will help to protect your brain from free-radicals. Follow the recommendations in Chapter 26 for dosage guidelines.

Vitamin B-complex is also essential for healthy brain function. Some of the same factors that are associated with cardiovascular disease, such as elevated homocysteine levels, are also linked to decreased brain function. Taking a high-potency B-complex vitamin daily that includes 100 milligrams of vitamin B-6 and at least 400 micrograms of folic acid will help to prevent the accumulation of dangerous homocysteine in your bloodstream. In addition, a lack of vitamin B-12 is dangerous for your mental functioning—it's not uncommon for a B-12 deficiency to be mistaken for senility. Deficiencies with aging are not unusual, because many women have diminished digestive function at midlife, which inhibits the absorption of vitamin B-12. In addition to a high-potency B-complex supplement, take an additional 1,000 micrograms of B-12 daily in the form of an easily absorbable supplement such as a sublingual tablet that is dissolved under the tongue, or a nasal spray. To improve your digestion and absorption, take an herbal digestive tonic before meals (see page 197).

Herbal Help for Mental Clarity

Several herbs are excellent for enhancing brain function. The following herbs are safe to take over a long period of time and can be thought of as "brain tonics." In fact, they work best when taken for at least three months or longer.

Ginkgo (*Ginkgo biloba)* is probably the best herb for improving mental functioning. Derived from the leaves of an ancient tree that dates back to prehistoric times, ginkgo has been used for centuries in China to improve brain function. It contains flavonoid compounds called ginkgo heterosides and terpene lactones that have potent antioxidant properties, enhance circulation, and inhibit dangerous blood clots that can lead to brain-damaging strokes. Ginkgo has been proven in numerous studies to improve symptoms of mental decline related to impaired blood flow to the brain such as memory loss, mental confusion, and difficulties in concentrating. Ginkgo has even been shown to be beneficial in many cases of senile dementia, including the early stages of Alzheimer's disease. Take an extract of ginkgo standardized to contain 24 percent ginkgo heterosides (ginkgo flavone glycosides), 80 milligrams three times a day.

Siberian ginseng *(Eleutherococcus senticosus)* is a tonic herb that helps the body to more easily adapt to physical, mental, and emotional stressors. It strengthens and balances the nervous system and provides a mild energy boost that helps to improve mental focus. In several studies, people taking Siberian ginseng demonstrated marked improvement on cognitive function tests, including an increased ability to concentrate, quicker reaction time, and improved memory. Take an extract standardized for eleutherosides, 250 milligrams twice daily. Siberian ginseng is best used cyclically, taking the herb for two months followed by a two-week break before resuming the dosage. If you have high blood pressure, consult your doctor before taking any type of ginseng.

Gotu kola *(Centella asiatica)* is an Indian herb that is considered to be an important rejuvenative tonic in Ayurvedic medicine for the brain and nerve cells. It has long been used in India as a brain tonic, where it is taken to increase intelligence and memory and to ward off senility. Because of its calming properties, gotu kola is believed to be one of the most spiritual of all herbs and is used to heighten awareness for meditation practices. Gotu kola is a pretty plant that is easily grown indoors. You can add several leaves to a salad daily, or take one-half teaspoon of extract in warm water three times a day.

If you simply want to preserve healthy mental functioning and are not suffering from memory loss, you can make your own herbal formula to use as a brain tonic. However, if you currently have noticeable memory loss or other symptoms of decreased cognitive functioning, it's best to take standardized extracts of ginkgo and Siberian ginseng, as described earlier.

Herbal Tonic for Mental Clarity

1 ounce ginkgo liquid extract

1 ounce Siberian ginseng liquid extract

1/2 ounce gotu kola liquid extract

Combine extracts in a dark-glass bottle, and store in a cool, dark place. Shake well before using, and take 1/2 teaspoon of extract in a small amount of warm water 3 times a day.

Essential Oils to Clear Mental Fatigue

Transient mental fogginess can be caused by overthinking, over-working, and fatigue. Essential oils can help to clear the mind, relieve fatigue, and sharpen your mental focus. *Rosemary* and *basil* are two of the best essential oils for stimulating brain function. Place a drop or two of either one (or a combination of both) on a handkerchief and inhale the fragrance as needed, or make the following air freshener to spray into the air when you need a boost of mental clarity.

Mental-Clarity Room Freshener

1 tablespoon witch hazel

10 drops rosemary essential oil

10 drops basil essential oil

5 drops lavender essential oil

2 cups water

Combine witch hazel and essential oils in a 16-ounce spray bottle and shake well. Add water to fill the bottle, shake thoroughly, and spray as desired into the air.

Lifestyle Suggestions for Improving Brain Function

The way you live on a daily basis has a great deal to do with how your brain functions today and how healthy your cognitive abilities will remain as you age. Make sure that you are getting enough sleep, because sufficient rest is necessary for your brain to function properly. Some of the primary symptoms of sleep deprivation are memory loss, difficulties concentrating, and impairment in cognitive abilities. If you have trouble sleeping, try taking a warm bath before bed with two cups of Epsom salts dissolved in the water; these are rich in magnesium and help to relax the body and the nervous system. Drinking a cup of *chamomile* or *passionflower* tea can also help to calm the mind and induce restful sleep. For more suggestions for treating insomnia, see Chapter 15.

As important as is proper rest, physical exercise is equally essential for healthy brain function. Aerobic exercise improves circulation, which increases the supply of oxygen and nutrients to your brain. Regular exercise also helps to prevent atherosclerosis, high blood pressure, and other degenerative diseases that contribute to impaired mental function. A daily walk is an excellent way to alleviate emotional stress. I find that there is nothing more effective than a brisk walk to clear my mind, which automatically results in sharper mental focus and a sense of calm that permeates my entire being. Yoga is also effective for cultivating mental clarity. The deep, rhythmical breathing and gentle stretching of yoga help to calm the body and mind, increase circulation, and bring renewed energy to the brain by enhancing oxygenation of the brain cells. Breathing exercises (called *pranayama)* have been used for centuries by yoga practitioners to cultivate increased mental clarity and focus. Try the following yoga breathing exercise to refresh your mind. In this exercise, the exhalation is forceful, sharp, and quick, while the inhalation is spontaneous, fluid, and easy.

ENERGIZING BREATH

1. Sit in a comfortable position with your spine straight and your shoulders relaxed.
2. Inhale and exhale slowly and deeply a few times through your nose to relax your body and mind and to establish a comfort-

able breathing rhythm. As you inhale, gently expand your abdomen, and as you exhale, gently contract your abdomen.

3. Exhale forcefully through your nose, at the same time drawing your abdominal muscles in toward your spine. Focus on expelling as much stale air from your lungs as possible during the exhalation.

4. Allow your inhalation to occur naturally by simply relaxing your abdomen immediately following the powerful exhalation.

5. Repeat in a steady rhythm for as long as you are comfortably able for up to one minute.

Just as you need to engage in physical exercise to keep your body strong, you need to engage in mental exercise to keep your mind strong. Intellectual activity stimulates the development of new connections between brain cells, which helps to balance the normal cellular deterioration that occurs with aging. Mental activities that help to keep your brain young include playing games such as word games or other games that require thinking, strategy, and recall. Get away from watching television, which is a passive activity and does little to challenge your brain cells. Instead, expand your mind by reading, attending cultural events, taking classes, engaging in interesting conversation, and traveling. Anything you do that challenges you to think in new ways encourages the growth of your mental abilities. In the same vein, trying new activities helps you to maintain interest in life, which keeps your brain out of a rut. Take time every day to do things that you enjoy doing and to be with people whom you find stimulating and interesting.

For optimal brain functioning, it is also essential to simply pay attention. Many times, forgetfulness is the result of going unconscious, of not paying attention to what you are doing in the present moment. The more closely you observe the details of daily life, the sharper you hone your mental focus. Meditation is a wonderful way of learning to stay in the present moment and also helps to lessen emotional stress, which inhibits mental functioning. Long-term stress has actually been found to damage brain cells in the hippocampus, the result of elevated levels of cortisol, a hormone secreted by the adrenal glands in response to stress. Experiment with meditation and relaxation practices to reduce stress in your life, and choose one that you feel comfortable with to practice daily (see Appendix II for suggestions).

Chapter 17

Control Hypoglycemia and Diabetes

Hypoglycemia and diabetes are common conditions that are primarily the result of an unhealthful diet and lifestyle. That's good news, because it means that in the vast majority of cases, modifying your diet and making a few lifestyle changes can stabilize or even reverse the disease process. Diabetes and hypoglycemia both involve problems with maintaining stable blood-sugar levels and most of the time are caused by the typical diet we have come to regard as normal—a diet loaded with refined carbohydrates and sweets.

The Dangers of Unstable Blood Sugar

The body requires blood-sugar levels to be in a fairly narrow range and accomplishes this through the combined efforts of the pancreas, adrenal glands, and liver. If something goes awry, however, and one or more of the supporting organs or glands is not functioning properly, disruptions in blood sugar can occur. Hypoglycemia is the result of blood-sugar levels that have fallen too low, while diabetes is a condition of blood-sugar levels that have risen to dangerously high levels.

For food to be used as fuel, it has to first be converted into glucose, or sugar. Glucose is the primary source of energy for the body and the brain, and for optimal health and energy, blood-sugar levels must remain in a normal range. The pancreas is the organ in charge of monitoring blood-sugar levels. During the process of digestion, glucose is released into the bloodstream, which triggers the pancreas to secrete the hormone insulin. Insulin stimulates cells to increase their uptake of glucose and returns blood-sugar levels to a normal range. When blood-sugar levels drop, which happens during exercise or if it has been several hours since eating a meal, the pancreas secretes another hormone called glucagon. Glucagon stimulates the liver to release glycogen, glucose that it has stored to provide the body and brain with an uninterrupted source of fuel. The adrenal glands also play an important role in managing blood-sugar levels. Emotional stress or rapid decreases in blood-sugar levels trigger the adrenals to release the hormone adrenaline, which increases the rate at which stored glucose is broken down to provide the body with the extra boost of energy it needs to adequately meet a crisis situation.

These blood-sugar regulating systems all work beautifully unless they are exhausted by high-sugar diets. When the pancreas, liver, and adrenals are overtaxed, hypoglycemia and diabetes are frequently the result. The reason that sugar is the primary culprit behind hypoglycemia and diabetes is that refined sugars are easily absorbed into the bloodstream, which causes blood-sugar levels to rapidly increase and begins a chain reaction of overstimulating the pancreas, liver, and adrenals as they each play their part in attempting to regulate blood-sugar levels. Hypoglycemia is usually the initial condition caused by high-sugar intake, but if the pancreas continues to be stressed, it becomes exhausted and stops producing insulin, or the cells themselves become insensitive to the effects of insulin. Either way, diabetes is the result.

Diagnosing Hypoglycemia

Hypoglycemia, commonly referred to as low blood sugar, occurs when the body is unable to maintain stable levels of glucose in the bloodstream. The symptoms of hypoglycemia range from mild to severe, and include food cravings (especially for sweets), fatigue, dizziness, mood swings, headaches, and mental fogginess. While it's normal to feel a bit tired or cranky if you haven't eaten for several hours, if your blood-sugar regulating organs and glands are working efficiently, eating will take care of the problem. Chronic hypoglycemia is different and is a signal that the pancreas and the adrenal glands are not functioning up to par and are having difficulty maintaining stable blood-sugar levels.

You can be tested for hypoglycemia with a glucose-tolerance test, which measures how well your body handles glucose. However, it's an unpleasant procedure that requires drinking an intensely sweet sugar solution and having your blood taken every hour for at least four hours.

Hypoglycemia Symptoms

The glucose tolerance test is often not an accurate measurement for hypoglycemia; a much simpler diagnostic tool is self-evaluation of your symptoms.

Cravings for sweets or carbohydrates

Fatigue or weakness

Irritability

Headaches

Dizziness

Heart palpitations

Shakiness

Cold sweats

Nausea

Blurred vision

Difficulty concentrating

Mood swings

Nervousness

If your symptoms appear approximately three hours after a meal (especially a meal that is primarily refined carbohydrates), then hypoglycemia is likely the cause. Some doctors maintain that hypo-glycemia is a normal reaction to the body needing fuel. It *is* normal to crave food and feel fatigued when your blood-sugar levels drop—that's how your body lets you know that you need food. But it's all a matter of degree, and while some women experience only mild symptoms that occur after going hours without food, others suffer daily from a variety of unpleasant and debilitating symptoms caused by low blood sugar. If you have symptoms of hypoglycemia, it is a definite indication that your body is having difficulty manag-ing blood-sugar levels. If you suspect that you have hypoglycemia, you have nothing to lose and everything to gain by adopting a healthful diet and lifestyle that will help to restore your organs and glands to healthy functioning.

How to Eat to Control Blood-Sugar Levels

Sugar is the primary culprit in the development of hypoglycemia and diabetes. While sugar does provide a temporary boost of ener-gy, eating it too frequently puts tremendous stress on the organs and glands that regulate blood-sugar levels. If you don't have hypo-glycemia or diabetes or if you rarely indulge in sugar, your pancreas can handle occasional sugary treats. But if you frequently eat sugar, your pancreas can become hypersensitive to sugar and overreact, flooding your body with insulin, which causes blood-sugar levels to plummet. This triggers your adrenal glands into action, and they notify your liver to release the glucose that it has stored as emer-gency fuel, which once again floods your bloodstream with sugar. If this happens too many times, your pancreas can finally give up and stop producing insulin or your cells may become resistant to insulin, and hypoglycemia can slip into diabetes.

Most American women eat about 80 pounds of sugar per year, as well as large amounts of refined carbohydrates such as white flour, which is easily converted into glucose in the body. Even if you don't add sugar to foods, you can still take in tremendous amounts if your diet contains a lot of prepared foods. Obviously, desserts and sweets are loaded with sugar, but other foods such as salad dress-ings, pasta sauces, and dry cereals also typically contain large amounts of sugar. Sugar is hidden in foods in many forms and is often used in more than one form in processed foods. To help restore healthy blood-sugar levels, avoid all forms of sugar, including sucrose, glucose, maltose, corn syrup, honey, maple syrup, barley malt, and molasses. Learn to enjoy the unprocessed sweetness of fresh fruits (in moderation) and sweet vegetables such as yams, carrots, and winter squash. Although giving up concentrated sweeteners may be difficult initially, you will find that your cravings for sugar will diminish within a few weeks.

Other foods that interfere with healthy blood-sugar levels include refined carbohydrates such as breads and pastas made from white flour and white rice, all of which are rapidly broken down into simple sugars in the body. Stimulants such as caffeine offer a temporary burst of energy, but stress the adrenal glands and further impair their ability to normalize blood-sugar levels. Alcohol also interferes with blood-sugar stability because it hinders the body's ability to use glucose and stimulates the release of insulin, which causes blood sugar take a nosedive.

To help maintain steady blood-sugar levels, eat a diet high in fiber, especially soluble fiber, which slows down the digestion and absorption of carbohydrates and prevents rapid increases in blood-sugar levels. Soluble fiber keeps the pancreas from secreting too much insulin by enhancing cell sensitivity to insulin and improves the use of glucose by the liver, which prevents blood-sugar levels from remaining too high. Strive for at least 35 grams and preferably 50 grams of fiber each day. Legumes, whole grains, nuts, seeds, vegetables, and fruits are good sources of fiber, and especially good sources of soluble fiber include legumes, oat bran, most vegetables, apples, and pears. Eat carbohydrates in as close to their natural state as possible, because the fiber content helps to slow the absorption of natural sugars that carbohydrates contain—for example, eat an apple instead of drinking apple juice. Psyllium-seed husks, guar gum, and pectin are excellent sources of supplemental soluble fiber. To help balance blood-sugar levels, take one to three teaspoons of a fiber supplement stirred into a glass of water twice daily before meals.

Protein is essential for the proper functioning of the adrenal glands, pancreas, and liver and prevents cravings for high-carbohydrate foods. Because protein does not stimulate the release of insulin as do carbohydrates, it helps to stabilize blood-sugar levels. For maximum blood-sugar stability, eat three to four ounces of protein at lunch and at dinner. Moderate amounts of healthful fats are also essential for helping to maintain healthy blood-sugar levels and for providing a feeling of satiety, which helps to reduce cravings for carbohydrates. Raw nuts and seeds, avocados, olive oil, and flaxseed oil are all good sources of health-enhancing fats.

Eating frequent small meals is a helpful strategy for stabilizing blood-sugar levels. Avoid skipping meals, or going for more than two to three hours without eating. Get into the habit of eating meals at regular times, because your body functions best on a regular schedule. Plan for three meals a day, plus midmorning, midafternoon, and evening snacks. Include a small amount of protein or fat in your snack to help keep blood sugar stable—for example, have an apple with a few almonds, crackers with tofu spread, or carrot sticks with a few walnuts.

Supplements that are especially helpful for balancing blood-sugar include chromium, a trace mineral that is essential for the proper functioning of insulin. Take 200 to 600 micrograms of chromium picolinate daily. To help strengthen the adrenal glands, take 2,000 milligrams of vitamin C daily in divided doses and a high-potency multivitamin and mineral that provides 50 to 100 milligrams of the B-complex vitamins.

Herbal Help for Hypoglycemia

The most important herb you can take to help keep your blood-sugar levels balanced is Siberian ginseng *(Eleutherococcus senticosus)*. This remarkable herb helps to increase the body's resistance to stress and is an excellent general-tonic herb. It strengthens the adrenal glands, increases energy, and helps to stabilize blood-sugar levels. For best results, take an extract standardized for eleutherosides, which are regarded as the primary active compounds. Take 250 milligrams for two months, with a two-week break before resuming the dosage.

An herbal tea made from *burdock root, dandelion root,* and *licorice root* can also help to regulate blood sugar levels. Burdock and dandelion both improve liver function, which helps to keep blood sugar levels stable. Licorice root nourishes and strengthens the adrenal glands and provides a natural sweetness that does not disrupt blood sugar. If you have hypertension, consult your health practitioner before using licorice root.

Blood Sugar Balancing Tea

1 tablespoon dandelion root
1 tablespoon burdock root
1 tablespoon licorice root

Bring herbs and 3 1/2 cups of water to boil over medium heat in a covered pot. Lower the heat and simmer gently for 15 minutes. Remove from heat and steep an additional 15 minutes. Strain, and drink 3 cups a day.

The Role of Exercise in Balancing Blood Sugar

Exercise is essential for maintaining healthy blood-sugar levels. Regular moderate exercise enhances the ability of cells to respond to insulin and to absorb glucose. The more fit you are, the more responsive your cells will be to insulin, which helps to keep blood sugar under control. Through its positive effect on blood-sugar levels, exercise helps to prevent diabetes. Exercising moderately and regularly is also extremely important if you have diabetes. Because exercise helps to decrease blood-glucose levels and enhances cellular response to insulin, it often lowers insulin requirements. Regular exercise has other benefits as well: It helps to decrease carbohydrate cravings, increases energy levels, and helps to prevent the common complications of diabetes such as cardiovascular disease and impaired circulation. Exercise also improves the health of the adrenal glands by defusing emotional stress, which is a primary cause of adrenal fatigue and a contributing factor to blood-sugar imbalances. Plan for at least 30 minutes of activity such as walking or biking at least five days a week.

How Diabetes Occurs

The incidence of diabetes is increasing every year and is now the fourth-leading cause of death in the United States. Symptoms of diabetes include increased thirst and urination, and weakness or fatigue. There are two different types of diabetes, labeled as insulin dependent or type I, and noninsulin dependent, or type II. Type I diabetes is thought to be a type of autoimmune disease that destroys the pancreatic cells. There is often a genetic predisposition, and the onset is frequently triggered in susceptible people by a bout with a viral infection such as the flu. Type I diabetics are dependent on insulin, which they must inject daily to control blood sugar.

Type II diabetes almost always appears after the age of 40, and 90 percent of the time is caused by years of accumulated damage to the blood-sugar regulating mechanisms of the body. Type II diabetics do produce insulin—sometimes even larger amounts than normal—but the cells are not able to use it properly. Risk factors for the onset of type-II diabetes include a high-sugar diet, smoking, obesity, and lack of exercise. Not surprisingly, diabetes is rarely found in cultures that eat a more traditional diet that excludes processed foods and refined sugars.

Diabetes occurs when the pancreas stops making insulin, or when the cells become unable to use the insulin that the pancreas produces. This means that the cells are unable to use food for energy, because insulin regulates the levels of glucose in the bloodstream. During the process of digestion, the liver processes carbohydrates, storing part as emergency fuel reserves and releasing the rest into the bloodstream as an immediate source of energy for the body. As levels of glucose increase, the pancreas is triggered to secrete insulin, which aids the cells in absorbing glucose. In diabetes, however, this process does not occur as it is meant to and blood sugar accumulates to dangerous levels in the bloodstream.

High concentrations of glucose in the blood create many problems, including the narrowing of small blood vessels throughout the body. This impairs circulation, which can cause serious complications such as slow wound healing, kidney disease, nerve degeneration, and eye disease that can progress to blindness. High levels of blood sugar also impair the way that fats are metabolized and increases the risk of atherosclerosis (hardening of the arteries) and heart disease.

Treating Diabetes Naturally

Type II diabetes is conventionally treated with drugs to stimulate insulin production and increase the insulin sensitivity of tissues. If those treatments fail to control blood sugar, insulin injections are prescribed. Side effects of the drugs used include hypoglycemia, immune suppression, headaches, fatigue, nausea, liver and kidney damage, and a greater risk of cardiovascular disease. In the majority of cases, drugs and insulin are not necessary for Type II diabetes, because the disease can be controlled—and sometimes even reversed—with dietary and lifestyle changes. *If you are interested in taking a natural approach to diabetes, do so under the supervision of your health care practitioner and closely monitor your blood sugar levels.*

Diet and lifestyle changes, including losing excess weight, are extremely successful in treating diabetes. Even if you suffer from Type I diabetes, the suggestions given here can help you manage your condition so that you can take the least amount of insulin necessary to maintain healthy blood-sugar levels. While it is essential to work closely with a health-care practitioner if you have diabetes, ultimately, the course of the condition is primarily up to you.

Pamela was diagnosed with diabetes at age 46. She had been feeling fatigued and noticed that she was constantly thirsty and urinating frequently, but she never suspected she had diabetes. She had suffered for years from hypoglycemia and had managed to survive attacks of low blood sugar by eating more sugar to boost her energy and by drinking coffee and colas throughout the day. The diagnosis of diabetes came as a shock, and because she didn't want to take drugs to control her blood-sugar levels, she was motivated to make changes in her life to try to get her blood sugar under control. She cut out sugar and caffeine, started eating small meals several times a day composed of complex carbohydrates, protein, and healthful fats, and began taking *gymnema sylvestre,* an herb that helps to control blood sugar. Even though she had never enjoyed exercise, she enlisted the help of friends to go for walks several mornings a week. In less than three months, Pamela's blood sugar was under control, she had lost 25 pounds, and she felt better than she had in years.

The diet-and-exercise suggestions given earlier for hypoglycemia are equally appropriate for treating diabetes. Pay special attention to consuming large amounts of soluble fiber. Eating legumes such as lentils, kidney beans, black beans, and other types of beans is especially helpful because they are rich in soluble fiber and are slowly digested, which releases small amounts of glucose into the bloodstream over a long period of time. Eat beans daily in the form of soups, stews, pasta dishes, and in salads. Include lots of garlic and onions in your diet, too, because they help to lower blood-sugar levels and increase levels of insulin in the bloodstream. Because diabetes is associated with a disturbance in essential-fatty-acid metabolism, supplementing with essential fatty acids is important. To obtain omega-3 fatty acids, eat cold-water fish such as salmon, sardines, halibut, and mackerel two to three times per week, and take one tablespoon of flaxseed oil daily. In addition, take supplements of gamma linolenic acid (GLA) in the form of evening primrose oil, black currant oil, or borage oil, 240 milligrams daily.

Herbal Help for Diabetes

The following herbs are especially helpful for both Type I and Type II diabetes.

Gymnema *(Gymnema sylvestre)* has long been used in Ayurvedic medicine to treat diabetes. It enhances the production of insulin by the pancreas, improves blood-sugar control, and helps to decrease blood sugar, trigylcerides, and cholesterol. Gymnema even appears to help regenerate the pancreas and is effective for both Type I and Type II diabetes. It has no harmful side effects, but if you are taking gymnema, be sure to tell your health-care practitioner because it can decrease your need for diabetic drugs. Take 200 milligrams twice a day.

Bilberry *(Vaccinium myrtillus)* is helpful for preventing and treating diabetic retinopathy, an eye condition common in diabetics that can cause blindness. Bilberry helps to strengthen the small blood vessels and prevents breakage. The active compounds in bilberry, called anthocyanosides, are especially beneficial for the blood vessels of the eye and improve circulation to the retina. Take between 80 and 160 milligrams of an extract standardized for 25 percent anthocyanidins three times per day.

Ginkgo *(Ginkgo biloba)* also helps to strengthen the blood vessels, making them more flexible and less likely to break. In addition, ginkgo improves blood flow to the extremities, making it very helpful for improving the poor circulation that often occurs with diabetes. Take an extract standardized for 24 percent ginkgo flavoglycosides, 40 to 80 milligrams three times per day.

Chapter 18

Relief for Varicose Veins

Varicose veins are extremely common, affecting almost one out of every four women. While they rarely present a serious health problem, the characteristically swollen, discolored, and distorted veins are often painful and unattractive. Rachel was in her early thirties when she first noticed tiny red spider veins on her thighs and on the insides of her ankles. Her legs ached, especially just prior to and during her menstrual cycle and at times, the aching was so uncomfortable that it kept her awake at night. She realized that she had the beginning symptoms of varicose veins, and in an effort to prevent them from growing worse Rachel started a program of daily walking and yoga to improve the circulation in her legs and began taking vitamin C to strengthen her veins. This worked fine until she reached her forties, but when her hormones started to fluctuate as she approached menopause, she began experiencing leg aches again as well as more spider veins and a few larger discolored surface veins. Rachel's mother had suffered from severe varicose veins and had resorted to surgery to remove the problem veins. Rachel was determined to do everything possible to avoid such drastic measures. She added herbs such as horse chestnut to improve her circulation and strengthen her veins, made an aromatherapy-massage oil to soothe her legs, and consciously changed habits such as sitting too long that contribute to the development of varicose veins. It took only about a month for Rachel to notice that the aching in her legs was easing, and after three months, she had no further symptoms.

How to Prevent Varicose Veins

The swollen, twisted, and discolored veins that are characteristic of varicose veins occur when blood pools in the legs and distorts the veins. Blood is returned to the heart via a network of veins throughout the body, and the veins in the legs have the difficult task of directing blood to flow uphill. A series of valves in the veins keeps the blood from flowing backwards, but the valves can be faulty for a variety of reasons. Varicose veins typically appear along the insides of the legs and the backs of the calves. Common symptoms include tired, aching legs and swollen ankles and feet. Often, the skin covering the veins becomes sensitive and itches. The swollen, twisted veins are usually surrounded by hard, lumpy tissue caused by an excess of fibrin, a protein made by the body that promotes blood clotting and the formation of scar tissue. Healthy veins naturally produce a substance that helps to break down excess fibrin, but people with varicose veins have a decreased ability to break down fibrin.

Many women find that their symptoms are worse before and during menstruation, and also in the perimenopausal years because high levels of estrogen weaken the veins. While most varicose veins occur on the surface of the legs, a more serious type are those that affect the deeper leg veins. These deep veins are more prone to inflammation, and blood clots can form on the vein walls. If blood clots break loose, they can travel to the lungs through the bloodstream and may cause serious damage. If you have painful leg swelling that does not diminish after elevating your legs, consult your physician immediately because it may signal a dangerous blood clot.

A variety of factors contribute to varicose veins, including an inherited tendency to have weak veins or valves. However, many cases of varicose veins are caused by factors that increase pressure in the legs, all of which you can prevent. Being overweight, standing or sitting for long periods of time, constipation, and tight clothing that restricts blood flow in the pelvis and legs all impair circulation and contribute to weakening the veins. Simple habits that you can cultivate to prevent varicose veins include avoiding sitting or standing for long periods of time. Make an effort to get up and move around every half hour if you are sitting, and if you must stand for any length of time, keep moving to prevent blood from pooling in your legs. The movement of leg muscles acts like a pump to push your blood up through your veins on its return journey to the heart.

Whenever possible, raise your legs while you are sitting to ease the workload on your veins. Place a small stool under your desk to elevate your feet, and use a footstool or a recliner at home. One of the best things you can do to prevent varicose veins and to relieve the symptoms of existing ones is to walk every day for at least 45 minutes. You might consider breaking the walk up into 15-minute segments in the morning, afternoon, and evening to give your circulation a significant boost three times a day. In addition to active exercise, take time every day to relax with your legs raised above your head to ease the pressure on your veins. Lie on your back on the floor near a wall, and place your feet on the wall so that your legs are at a 45-degree angle to your body. Relax for 10 to 15 minutes in this position one or more times daily.

Dietary Help for Strengthening Veins

The most important dietary factor for preventing and relieving varicose veins is fiber. Constipation is a primary cause of varicose veins because straining during bowel movements increases pressure in the abdomen and restricts blood flow through the pelvis and legs, which over time weakens the vein walls. Eating a high-fiber diet is easy if you make a conscious effort to eat plenty of fresh vegetables, fruits, whole grains, legumes, nuts, and seeds. Supplemental fiber in the form of psyllium husks can also be helpful. Each morning, take one to three teaspoons of powdered psyllium husks stirred into one-half glass of water or juice, followed by an additional glass of water.

Foods that are especially helpful for varicose veins include those that are rich in anthocyanidins, the substance that gives cherries, blueberries, blackberries, and purple grapes their deep blue-red color. Anthocyanidins strengthen the veins and the connective tissue that supports the blood vessels and help to prevent blood from leaking through fragile capillary walls. Eat at least one cup of these health-promoting fruits daily. Other foods that have a positive effect on varicose veins are garlic, onions, ginger, and cayenne. These spicy foods help the body to break down fibrin, the protein that creates hard, lumpy tissue surrounding varicose veins. Include liberal amounts of these healthful foods in your cooking to spice up your meals and at the same time to improve the health of your veins.

Supplements that are especially helpful for preventing and relieving varicose veins include vitamin C and bioflavonoids, which help to strengthen veins and decrease capillary fragility. Take 1,000–2,000 milligrams of vitamin C combined with bioflavonoids daily in divided doses throughout the day. Grapeseed extract is an especially rich source of proanthocyanidins, another natural plant compound that strengthens veins and capillaries and increases the muscle tone of veins, improving their ability to contract and to move blood efficiently. Take between 150 and 300 milligrams of a standardized grapeseed extract daily. Vitamin E helps to improve circulation and also improves vein health. Take 800 units of vitamin E in the natural form of d-alpha tocopherol daily. Bromelain, a protein-digesting enzyme derived from pineapple stems, is helpful for breaking down fibrin. Take 500 milligrams two to three times a day. For dissolving fibrin, take bromelain separate from meals, because if it is taken with meals it will act as a digestive aid.

Herbal Relief for Varicose Veins

Herbs can be of great benefit for preventing and treating varicose veins. They increase circulation, strengthen blood vessels, and improve muscle tone in the vein walls, which enhances blood flow. Following are some of the most important herbs for treating varicose veins:

Horse chestnut *(Aesculus hippocastanum)* has been shown to be as effective as conventional treatments such as compression stockings for relieving the symptoms of varicose veins. The fruit of the horse chestnut tree has anti-inflammatory properties, helps to relieve leg swelling, and strengthens capillary walls. It enhances vascular tone by tightening the elastic fibers in vein walls, which improves blood flow and prevents blood from pooling in the legs. Scientists have identified the active ingredient in horse chestnut as aescin. For best results, take extracts that provide 50 milligrams of aescin twice daily. Do not exceed the recommended dosage, because while horse chestnut is safe, in larger amounts it can cause nausea, vomiting, and other unpleasant side effects.

Gotu kola *(Centella asiatica)* is an herb that has long been used in India for treating varicose veins. It strengthens the connective tissue that surrounds the vein, improves blood flow, and reduces hardening of the vein. In addition, gotu kola relieves the uncomfortable symptoms of varicose veins such as leg cramps, swelling, and feelings of heaviness in the legs. Take one-half teaspoon of gotu kola extract or two capsules three times a day.

Hawthorne *(Crataegus oxycantha)* is an excellent herb for any type of circulatory problem. It improves circulation and helps to relieve the fluid retention that may accompany varicose veins. The deep-blue-red hawthorne berries and flowers are also rich sources of anthocyanidins, the compounds that help to strengthen blood vessels. Hawthorne is a gentle, safe herb and is most effective when used over a long period of time. Make a tea by pouring one cup of water over two teaspoons of the crushed berries or flowers and leaves, cover, and steep for 20 minutes. Strain, and drink three cups a day. You can also take one-half teaspoon of liquid extract or two capsules three times a day.

Herbal Tea for Varicose Veins

2 teaspoons hawthorne berries or flowers
1 teaspoon grated fresh ginger root
1 cup water

Pour boiling water over herbs. Cover, and steep for 20 minutes. Strain, sweeten if desired, and drink 3 cups daily.

Ease Discomfort with Aromatherapy Oils

Combining hydrotherapy with therapeutic essential oils can effectively relieve the uncomfortable symptoms of varicose veins. Alternating hot and cold footbaths, compresses, and gentle massage help to relieve pain and aching and improve circulation, while cold compresses help to relieve inflammation and swelling. The following essential oils are especially useful for treating varicose veins.

Cypress has astringent and vein-tightening properties and stimulates circulation. It also helps to relieve fluid retention. Cypress has a spicy, pinelike fragrance.

Frankincense has anti-inflammatory and astringent properties, helps to tighten veins, and stimulates skin healing. It has a rich, warm, balsamic fragrance.

Yarrow contains azulene, a powerful natural anti-inflammatory that gives the essential oil a dark-blue color. The astringent properties of yarrow also help to tighten varicose veins. It has a fresh, herbaceous, pungent fragrance.

Varicose-Vein Massage Oil

4 ounces calendula infused oil (see recipe page 10) or almond oil

20 drops cypress essential oil

10 drops frankincense essential oil

10 drops yarrow essential oil

1 teaspoon vitamin E oil

Combine oils in a dark-glass bottle and shake thoroughly to mix. Store in a cool, dark place. Shake well before using. To use as a massage oil, apply approximately 1 teaspoon of oil to each leg with long, gentle strokes, always working from the foot up the leg in the direction of the heart.

Soothing Lotion for Varicose Veins

---

4 ounces distilled witch hazel

10 drops cypress essential oil

10 drops frankincense essential oil

Combine essential oils with witch hazel in a dark-glass bottle. Shake well. Apply to legs as often as desired. For additional pain-relieving effects, store the lotion in the refrigerator and apply cold to the legs.

Healing Footbath for Varicose Veins

Alternating hot and cold footbaths are excellent for both preventing the development of varicose veins and easing the pain and discomfort of existing ones. You'll need two plastic basins large enough to hold your feet. Fill one basin with water as hot as you can tolerate, and fill the other with cold water to which you have added a few ice cubes. Add five drops of cypress essential oil to the basin of hot water, sit in a comfortable chair, and slowly immerse your feet in the water. Leave your feet in the hot water for three minutes, and then immediately plunge your feet into the basin of cold water for one minute. Alternate back and forth between the hot and cold water three to five times, ending with the cold water. Finish by patting your feet dry and massaging your legs with the varicose-vein massage oil.

Chapter 19

Banish Migraine and Tension Headaches

Everyone experiences at least an occasional headache, and chronic headache pain plagues millions of women. By far the two most common types of headaches are tension headaches and vascular, or migraine headaches. Tension headaches arise from tense muscles in the head, face, and neck. Symptoms include tightness or soreness in the back of the neck and generalized pain, pressure, or aching throughout the head. Many women suffer from chronic tension headaches that last anywhere from a few minutes to a few days.

The intense debilitating pain of migraine headaches afflicts one out of every four women. Migraines are often severe and cause intense, sharp, throbbing pain that is usually localized to one side of the head. These headaches are often preceded by a feeling of anxiety or depression, numbness or tingling on one side of the body, and visual disturbances called "auras" that appear as flashing lights, blurred vision, or tunnel vision. Migraines can last from a few hours to a few days, and the pain can be incapacitating. Most researchers believe that migraines are caused by the constriction of blood vessels in the brain, followed by a sudden expansion of the vessels. There are many triggers for migraine headaches, including food allergies, chemical exposure, emotional tension, weather changes, and too little or too much sleep. Because hormonal fluctuations are also a primary contributing factor, women are three times more likely to suffer from migraines than are men.

Most people don't think twice about reaching for a pain-relieving drug to treat a headache, but researchers have found that the drugs commonly used for headaches, including analgesics such as aspirin or acetaminophen, are actually a contributing factor to chronic headaches, particularly for people who use them often. A much better alternative is to learn how to prevent headaches and to use natural, nontoxic herbs as needed for pain relief. Always consult your doctor if you experience an unusually severe headache, if a headache is accompanied by a fever of 102 degrees or higher, or if a headache lasts longer than three days.

A Nutritional Approach to Preventing Headaches

What you eat—and don't eat—plays an important role in preventing headaches. Avoiding caffeine and headache "trigger" foods is crucial. Caffeine is a powerful drug and is a primary factor in both tension and migraine headaches because it constricts blood vessels and contributes to overall physical and emotional tension. Avoid caffeine in all of its forms, including coffee, black tea, cola, chocolate, coffee and cocoa-flavored foods, and over-the-counter drugs that contain caffeine. If you currently use caffeine, giving it up will improve your health, but you will probably have severe withdrawal headaches for several days if you eliminate it suddenly. Taking a more gradual approach of cutting back on your intake of caffeine over a couple of weeks gives your body the opportunity to adjust without undue trauma. Try ginger tea, green tea, or an herbal tea with Siberian ginseng as a replacement for caffeinated drinks. These herbal beverages are beneficial for your health and provide a gentle energy boost without the negative drawbacks of caffeine.

Foods known to be triggers for migraine headaches include aged cheeses, beer, alcohol (especially red wine), chocolate, pickles, cured meats, and foods containing monosodium glutamate, nitrates, and artificial sweeteners. These foods contain substances that cause the blood vessels in the brain to expand, which sets the stage for a migraine. Many other foods, such as avocados, potatoes, shellfish, bananas, yeasted bread, and tomatoes can also cause migraines. Randomly trying to figure out what you can safely eat can be difficult, and there is no reason to unnecessarily restrict your diet. The best way to discover your migraine triggers is to keep a food-and-headache diary for a couple of weeks. Write down everything you eat, and also make a note of when you have headaches. With some diligence you should be able to see a correlation between your headaches and any dietary triggers.

Keeping your blood-sugar levels balanced is also important, because one of the most common symptoms that occurs when blood-sugar drops is a headache. Eat small, frequent meals every three hours, and avoid refined carbohydrates and sugars. High-protein foods and foods rich in complex carbohydrates along with moderate amounts of healthful fats are the best foods for helping to keep blood-sugar levels stable. See Chapter 17 for a thorough discussion of low blood sugar and treatment recommendations.

As with many inflammatory pain disorders, eating foods rich in omega-3 fatty acids has been found to reduce the incidence of migraine headaches by shifting the balance of hormone-like prostaglandins in favor of those that have anti-inflammatory, pain-relieving action and by decreasing inflammatory prostaglandins. Omega-3 fatty acids are found in cold-water fish (salmon, mackerel, and sardines), walnuts, flaxseeds, and flaxseed oil. Eat fish two or three times a week and take one tablespoon of flaxseed oil daily. Supplementing your diet with magnesium can also be helpful for preventing headaches. Magnesium is an excellent muscle and nerve relaxant and helps to keep blood vessels healthy. Take 250 milligrams of magnesium three times a day in the form of citrate, malate, or aspartate, which are easily absorbable forms of magnesium.

Regular exercise is also helpful for preventing the accumulation of emotional and physical tension. Many times, a tension headache can be relieved by going out for a brisk walk, which relieves muscle tension, increases circulation, and brings a fresh supply of oxygen to the brain. Sitting for too long causes energy to stagnate and contributes to muscle tension. Take time throughout the day for a few simple stretching exercises combined with deep breathing to keep your energy flowing, and plan a 30-minute walk or other form of enjoyable gentle moderate exercise five days a week or more.

Herbal Remedies for Headaches

The simple act of brewing and drinking a cup of hot herbal tea can do much to promote relaxation and relieve a tension headache, especially if it is made from a relaxing herb such as *chamomile, catnip,* or *linden flower,* all of which are mild sedatives. A more tenacious headache may require *white willow bark, meadowsweet,* or *valerian,* all of which have pain-relieving properties. These herbs generally do not work as well as drugs for stopping pain, but because they have no harmful side effects, they are a much better alternative. With migraines, herbs work best when used as preventative medicine.

Feverfew *(Tanacetum parthenium)* is a pretty, daisy-like herb that has been proven to reduce the number and severity of migraine attacks when taken regularly. The leaves of feverfew contain an active ingredient called parthenolide, which inhibits the production of substances that dilate blood vessels and cause inflammation. Feverfew is easy to grow, and migraine sufferers have reported relief from eating two of the fresh leaves daily. Feverfew is extremely bitter and can cause mouth or tongue irritation. To avoid this problem, try eating the leaves wrapped in a piece of fresh bread. You can also buy feverfew capsules or extract standardized for the active ingredient parthenolide. Take between one-quarter and one-half milligrams of parthenolide daily for migraine prevention, and up to two grams during an acute attack.

Ginger *(Zingiber officinalis)* also has potent anti-inflammatory properties and when eaten regularly can help to prevent migraines. Ginger improves circulation, relaxes the blood vessels, and decreases the production of pain-causing prostaglandins. Fresh ginger may be the most effective form of the herb for preventing migraines, because the pungent oils in the raw herb have the most active properties. For headache prevention, eat one-quarter inch slice of fresh ginger root daily, either raw or lightly cooked. If you prefer using dried ginger, buy good-quality powdered ginger and take 1,000 milligrams daily. In the event of a migraine, take 500 to 1,000 milligrams at the first sign and repeat every couple of hours up to six times a day as needed.

Migraine-Headache Formula

1 ounce feverfew extract
1/2 ounce chamomile extract
1/2 ounce ginger root extract

Combine extracts in a dark-glass bottle. Take 1/2 teaspoon in a small amount of warm water 2 times a day to prevent migraines, and up to every 2 hours at the onset of a migraine.

Tension-Headache-Relief Tea

2 teaspoons grated ginger root
2 teaspoons linden blossom
2 teaspoons chamomile
2 cups water

Simmer ginger root in water in a covered pot for 10 minutes. Remove from heat, add linden and chamomile, cover, and steep for 10 minutes. Strain, sweeten if desired, and drink hot as needed.

Relieve Headaches with Aromatherapy

Fragrant essential oils help to relieve headaches by easing mental and physical tension. The following essential oils are some of the most helpful for headaches.

Lavender is balancing for the body and mind and promotes relaxation. It relieves physical and mental stress and engenders an overall sense of well-being. Lavender has a sweet, floral, herbaceous fragrance.

Marjoram has potent sedative properties and is especially helpful for migraine headaches. It has a sweet, spicy, herbaceous scent.

Chamomile has anti-inflammatory and pain-relieving properties, helps to ease emotional tension, and is especially helpful for tension headaches. Chamomile has a sweet, herbaceous and slightly tart fragrance.

Peppermint helps to relieve pain, is antispasmodic, and stimulates circulation. The pungent menthol scent has an uplifting effect on the emotions and helps to clear the brain. Use in moderation.

Aromatherapy Compress for Tension Headaches

8 drops lavender essential oil
2 drops peppermint essential oil
2 cups cool water

Add essential oils to a basin of cool water. Soak two washcloths in the water, wring out, and apply one to the forehead and one to the back of the neck. Lie down and rest for 15 minutes or longer.

Aromatherapy Compress for Migraine Headaches

5 drops lavender essential oil
5 drops marjoram essential oil
2 cups cool water

Add essential oils to a basin of cool water. Soak two washcloths in the water, wring out, and apply one to the forehead and one to the back of the neck. Lie down and rest for 30 minutes or longer.

Massage Away Pain

Massage is a powerful technique for relaxing the tense muscles that contribute to headaches. By stimulating pressure points in the head and neck, you can release the blocked energy that causes tension and migraine headaches. You can easily massage your own temples, forehead, and neck, but you will have a more relaxing experience if someone else performs the massage on you.

The two points located just under the base of the skull where the neck joins the head are among the most important acupressure points for the head. To find these points, place your fingers at the top vertebrae of your neck, and then move your fingers to the side approximately one inch along the base of your skull until you feel a small indentation on either side. These points may feel slightly tender. Apply firm pressure with your thumbs or the pads of your fingers, making a small rotating motion if you desire. In general, the more deeply you massage the points, the better the results. Continue massaging for one to three minutes, until you feel the tension release from your neck and head.

Aromatherapy Massage Oil for Headaches

2 ounces almond oil
10 drops lavender essential oil
5 drops marjoram essential oil
5 drops chamomile essential oil
1/2 teaspoon vitamin E oil

Combine oils in a dark-glass bottle and shake well. Use approximately 1/2 teaspoon at a time and apply to the temples, forehead, back of the neck, and shoulders, massaging deeply to release blocked energy.

Hydrotherapy Treatments for Headaches

Hydrotherapy combined with aromatherapy is often effective for relieving headache pain. Soaking your hands in hot water at the first sign of a migraine helps to regulate circulation and can avert a full-blown migraine episode. Adding an essential oil such as marjoram or lavender to the hand bath makes the treatment even more effective. Add 10 drops of either essential oil (or a combination of the two) to a basin of hot water. Relax, breathe deeply, and soak your hands in the water for 15 minutes.

A hot footbath is excellent for easing a tension headache. Fill a basin with water as hot as you can comfortably tolerate, and add ten drops of lavender essential oil. Soak your feet in the hot water, and at the same time, place a cold cloth on the back of your neck or your forehead or wherever the pain is concentrated. Relax for at least 15 minutes, replacing the cold cloth with a fresh cloth as needed to maintain a cold temperature.

Relaxation for Headache Prevention

One of the most important things you can do to prevent headaches is to learn to relax. Taking the time to learn and practice relaxation techniques will give you the understanding of how you hold tension in your body and will give you the ability to recognize and let go of tension before it can accumulate. Practice the relaxation exercises in Appendix II, and consider biofeedback training if you suffer from chronic tension headaches or migraines. Biofeedback teaches you to become aware of what are normally unconscious and involuntary physiological responses, such as muscle tension and the constriction of circulation that causes migraines.

Chapter 20

Hints for Healthy Digestion

Even if you eat well and take supplements, you won't be healthy unless your digestion is optimal. The old adage, "You are what you eat" is true, but only if your body is absorbing the nutrients you take in and efficiently eliminating wastes. For most women, digestive functions typically begin to slow down after the age of 40. The stomach secretes less hydrochloric acid, the pancreas and small intestine make fewer digestive enzymes, and the liver becomes less efficient at metabolizing fats and sugars. But even though digestion may be less efficient at midlife and beyond, many digestive disturbances are caused by overeating, not eating enough fiber, eating while emotionally tense, or by eating foods that are difficult for the digestive system to handle, for example, fried foods, sweets, or red meats.

Gas, bloating, and feeling uncomfortably full after a meal are all signs that digestion is not up to par. Poor digestion can cause dry skin and hair, soft nails, and hair loss, and may also cause or contribute to more serious health conditions such as diverticulosis, heart disease, osteoporosis, lowered immunity, and varicose veins.

Simple Steps to Improve Digestion

One of the most important ways you can improve your digestion is to chew your food well. This may sound simplistic, but your stomach doesn't have teeth, and the more thoroughly you chew, the easier it is for your body to access nutrients from the foods that you eat. A good rule of thumb is to chew every mouthful of food until it is thoroughly pulverized. Drinking large amounts of fluids with meals can interfere with digestion and cause bloating, but sipping a small amount of liquid with your meal can enhance digestive function. A cup of *ginger, chamomile,* or *mint* herbal tea is an excellent digestive aid. Avoid eating when you are emotionally tense, because stress shuts down digestive processes. Make it a habit to take a couple of minutes to relax and slow down before eating. Take a couple of deep breaths, give your full attention to the food you are about to eat, and express your gratitude in whatever way feels comfortable to you for the nourishment you are about to receive.

For optimal digestive function, follow the dietary guidelines in Chapter 26. But note that even if you are eating a nutritious diet, you may suffer from digestive disturbances if the foods you are consuming are not healthful for your individual body chemistry. Food sensitivities often make their appearance at midlife as a result of diminished digestive enzymes and hydrochloric acid, the cumulative effect of years of dietary excesses, and long-term exposure to foods that are common allergens. Many women find at midlife that they are sensitive to foods that never bothered them when they were younger, for example, dairy products and wheat. Eliminating or cutting back on foods you are sensitive to can relieve digestive problems such as constipation, diarrhea, and indigestion, and may also help to ease PMS or menopausal symptoms of fatigue, depression, and irritability.

Identifying Problem-Causing Foods

Many digestive problems can be resolved simply by eliminating the foods that are taxing your digestive system. If every time you eat ice cream you get diarrhea, then you know clearly that ice cream is a problem for you. But unfortunately, the process of identifying problematic foods is not often so straightforward. Limiting your diet for a short period of time to foods that are not likely to cause food sensitivities can help to cleanse your body so that you can more easily identify troublesome foods. For ten days, eat only rice, quinoa, millet, fish, chicken, and vegetables, and cook with olive oil. For the first three days, you may find that you feel worse, because it takes time for the foods that might be causing problems to be eliminated from your body. After the first three days, however, most women find that they feel significantly better.

At the completion of the ten-day cleansing diet, add foods back into your diet one at a time to identify those that might be causing problems. Reintroduce one food every two days, eating the food twice each day to provide ample opportunity for any negative reaction to occur. During this process, keep a detailed daily journal and record all foods eaten as well as your energy levels and physical and emotional symptoms. If you discover that a particular food causes symptoms, eliminate that food for one month, and then try it again. Many foods that cause problems when eaten on a daily basis can be eaten occasionally without causing symptoms. Of course, it's important to not stress your digestion with foods that are detrimental to your health, such as high-fat, high-sugar, processed foods, and caffeine. Many women eat the same foods day after day, which increases the possibility of developing food sensitivities. Naturopathic doctors often recommend eating a simple rotation diet that involves not eating the same food more than once every four days. For example, if you eat wheat on Monday (including bread, pasta, and any other products made with wheat), then you would not eat it again until Friday. Eating a rotation diet has the additional benefit of encouraging you to branch out and to experiment with a variety of foods that will provide your body with a wide range of nutrients.

Make an Herbal Digestive Tonic to Enhance Digestion

Along with eating a balanced diet that is right for your particular body (see the suggestions in Chapter 26 for guidelines for a health-enhancing diet), you can enhance your digestive function with an *herbal-bitters tonic.* Herbs with bitter properties such as *dandelion root* and *gentian root* have been used for centuries by traditional cultures to encourage healthy digestion. Herbs with a bitter taste improve digestion by stimulating the digestive secretions and activities of the salivary glands, stomach, small intestine, gall bladder, and pancreas. All of this takes place when the bitter flavor comes into contact with taste receptors on the back of your tongue, which signal the central nervous system to set digestive processes in action.

A lack of the bitter taste in the modern diet is a primary contributing factor to poor digestion. While the flavors of sweet, salty, and sour are well represented in most women's diets, the bitter taste is one that is usually in short supply. Considering the many health benefits attributed to bitter foods and herbs, it's well worth cultivating an appreciation for bitter foods. Leafy greens are an excellent source of the bitter flavor—add arugula, watercress, or endive to your salads, or sauté mustard greens or dandelion greens as a side dish. It takes only a small amount of the bitter flavor to stimulate digestive function. In addition to including bitter foods in your diet, many women find that taking an herbal-bitters tonic is a helpful digestive aid, particularly if taken before meals containing fat or protein. Unlike supplements of digestive enzymes, bitter-herbal tonics do not make your digestive system lazy—on the contrary, when taken consistently, they actually nourish and support the functioning of the digestive organs.

The ideal time to take a bitters tonic is 10 to 20 minutes before a meal. Place one dropperful (about 30 drops) directly on your tongue or dilute the same dosage (about one-half teaspoon) in a small amount of warm water. Remember that to get your digestive juices flowing, the bitter taste needs to come into direct contact with your tongue. You can buy herbal-bitters tonics, or make your own with the following recipe.

Herbal Digestive Tonic

1/2 ounce dandelion root
1/4 ounce gentian root
1/4 ounce licorice root
1/4 ounce fennel seeds
1/4 ounce dried ginger root
1/4 ounce dried organic orange peel
1/4 ounce cardamom pods
vodka

1. *Using dried herbs, grind the herbs in a blender. Place in a glass jar and add enough vodka to cover the herbs, plus 2 inches. Close the jar tightly.*

2. *Place in a warm, dark place, and give the jar a gentle shake every day or two to keep the herbs from settling.*

3. *After 3 weeks, strain the liquid from the herbs through a strainer lined with several layers of cheesecloth, reserving the liquid. Squeeze the herbs to strain out all the liquid.*

4. *Funnel your bitters tonic into a dark-glass container, and store in a cool, dark place.*

Mild herbal teas that improve digestion include *chamomile, peppermint,* and *fennel,* all of which help to stimulate digestion and relieve gas. Try sipping the following tea after meals as a digestive aid.

Herbal Digestive Tea

1 teaspoon chamomile
1/2 teaspoon peppermint
1/2 teaspoon fennel seeds, crushed
1 cup water

Pour 1 cup boiling water over herbs. Cover, and let steep for 10 minutes. Strain, sweeten if desired, and drink while warm.

Ginger is a wonderful tonic herb for the digestive system. It contains essential oils that stimulate the production of digestive enzymes and helps to relieve heartburn, intestinal gas, and nausea. According to Ayurvedic medicine, ginger is excellent for stimulating *agni,* the digestive fire. It also helps to reduce *ama,* the accumulation of toxins in the digestive tract. Use ginger liberally in your cooking, and sip hot ginger tea during or after meals as a digestive aid.

Sweet-and-Spicy Ginger Tea

3–4 teaspoons chopped fresh ginger root

1 teaspoon fennel seeds

1 teaspoon licorice root

2 cups water

Place herbs in a pot with water and simmer, covered, for 10 minutes. Strain and drink as desired.

Relieve Constipation Naturally

Healthy digestion requires not only good assimilation of nutrients, but also the efficient elimination of wastes. Many women experience constipation at midlife, brought on by the slowing of digestive functions, poor eating habits, and lack of exercise. Bad breath, skin outbreaks, headaches, fatigue, and increased risk of intestinal and breast cancer are all related to chronically sluggish intestines. The regular use of any type of laxative—even herbal—can create dependence. Instead, address the root cause of constipation and your problems will be cured.

Eat a diet rich in fiber, which is easy to do if you consume plenty of vegetables, fruits, whole grains, legumes, nuts, and seeds every day. Fiber is the indigestible part of plants and acts as an intestinal broom by increasing the frequency and amount of bowel movements. Because fiber moves wastes quickly out of the body, it prevents toxins from being reabsorbed into the bloodstream. Another way that fiber helps to relieve constipation is by encouraging the growth of beneficial bacteria in the colon. In addition to eating high-fiber foods, you may find that your intestines work more efficiently when you include a fiber supplement in your diet. Psyllium-seed husks and pectin are excellent sources of supplemental fiber. Take one to three teaspoons of either once or twice daily with a large glass of water. If you have sensitive digestion, start with a small amount, perhaps one-half teaspoon, and gradually increase the amount over a period of several weeks until you are taking enough to produce the results you desire. Pay special attention to drinking plenty of fluids, at least six to eight glasses of pure water every day. Dehydration is a common and often overlooked cause of constipation.

An inadequate population of friendly intestinal bacteria is frequently an underlying cause of constipation and other digestive disturbances. Antibiotics, a diet high in sugar and processed foods, and low levels of digestive enzymes and stomach acids disrupt the body's internal ecology by reducing beneficial flora and promoting the overgrowth of troublesome microorganisms such as *Candida albicans.* Dietary supplements of *Lactobacillus acidophilus* and *Bactobacillus bifidum,* the friendly flora that normally inhabit the intestinal tract, can help to restore a healthy intestinal environment. Take supplements that provide at least one billion live microorganisms daily on an empty stomach before breakfast for at least one month. Supplements of beneficial flora are safe to use indefinitely and can be thought of more as concentrated foods than as supplements. Eating one cup of yogurt daily that contains live beneficial organisms is another way of nourishing friendly flora in the intestinal tract.

If you do occasionally need a laxative to get things moving, try the following herbal tea. *Cascara sagrada* is a gentle yet effective herbal stimulant laxative. *Licorice* soothes the intestinal tract and also has mild laxative properties, and *ginger root* and *fennel seed* help to prevent intestinal cramping.

Gentle Herbal Laxative Tea

---

1 teaspoon cascara sagrada bark
1/2 teaspoon licorice root
1/2 teaspoon ginger root
1/2 teaspoon fennel seed
1 cup water

Place herbs and water in a covered pot. Bring to a boil, remove from heat, and steep covered for 10 minutes. Strain, and drink before bed. If necessary, drink an additional cup in the morning.

Improve Digestion with Exercise and Massage

Regular daily exercise is essential for healthy digestive function. Aerobic exercise stimulates peristalsis, the movement of wastes through the large intestine, and also relieves the emotional tension that contributes to poor digestion. Walking is one of the best exercises for encouraging peristalsis. Try to walk for at least 30 minutes five days a week, and preferably every day. Yoga is also beneficial for enhancing digestive function and relieving constipation. When practiced regularly, the Half-Locust is an especially helpful yoga pose for improving digestive function.

THE HALF-LOCUST

- Lie on your stomach with your legs extended. Point your toes away from your body and place your chin on the floor.
- Place your arms alongside your body with your palms on the floor.
- Inhale, and stretch your right leg straight out behind your body. Lift your leg as high as you comfortably can without rolling to the side, and hold for a count of 10.
- Exhale, and lower your leg slowly to the floor. Repeat to the left side.
- Repeat the entire sequence 3 to 5 times.

A simple abdominal massage also improves intestinal function and stimulates the movement of wastes through the large intestine. This massage can be performed daily, preferably first thing in the morning before eating. Lie down and massage approximately one teaspoon of almond or olive oil onto your abdomen area (add two drops of marjoram essential oil if desired—it has gentle laxative properties). Starting at the lower right side of your abdomen, place your fingers flat against your abdomen and make small circular motions with your fingers. Press into your abdomen as deeply as you comfortably can. Using slow, circular movements, massage up the right side of your abdomen, across the center just above your navel, and down the left side, following the path of the large intestine. Make several circuits of your abdomen, and finish by rubbing your abdomen with the palms of your hands in the same clockwise direction, using smooth, gliding strokes.

Chapter 21

Maintain Strong Bones

Osteoporosis is the most common health problem for postmenopausal women—more common than cardiovascular disease, diabetes, arthritis, or breast cancer. At least one of every four postmenopausal women has osteoporosis, and more than 45,000 women die each year from osteoporosis-related injuries such as fractures of the hip and spine. Although the effects of osteoporosis are not likely to show up until a woman is in her sixties or seventies, bone loss actually begins decades earlier. Bone deterioration and fragility are not inevitable, however. Even if you have been diagnosed with osteoporosis, there is much that you can do to strengthen your bones and prevent further bone loss.

The Hidden Danger of Osteoporosis

Osteoporosis literally means "porous bones." Although bone seems to be rigid and dense, it is actually active,

living tissue. Your body is continually breaking down and rebuild-
ing bone tissue in a process called remodeling. The bones are a
storehouse for calcium, a mineral that is used for many essential
metabolic functions. Calcium is necessary not only for strengthening
bones and teeth, but it is also critical for regulating muscle contractions (including heartbeat), transmission of nerve impulses, and
blood clotting. Various glands regulate calcium levels in the bloodstream and pull it out of the bones when it is needed. Calcium is so
essential to our well-being that even a small variation in blood levels can be dangerous. For this reason, the concentration of calcium
in the blood is closely monitored and maintained within narrow limits by the parathyroid and thyroid glands, which ensure that an adequate amount is circulating in the bloodstream at all times. When
more calcium is needed by the body, cells that break down bone
(osteoclasts) step up their activity, calcium absorption in the intestinal tract is increased, and the kidneys decrease their excretion of
calcium. These calcium-preserving measures are triggered by a diet
that is too low in calcium and by a sedentary lifestyle. Fortunately,
calcium can also be put back into the bones. Physical work and
exercise demand stronger bones, and if the diet is calcium rich, calcium is deposited from the bloodstream into the bones.

Most bone building takes place in youth and early adulthood,
with a woman achieving her peak bone strength when she is in her
twenties. Ideally, regular daily exercise and optimal nutrition in
these formative years will build a strong skeletal structure that will
carry a woman into a healthy old age. But many women entering
menopause today did not have the benefit of this knowledge in
their younger years, and their diets were less than ideal and exercise was not a priority. Entering the menopausal years with less than
optimal bone mass means that more attention needs to be paid to
diet and exercise to prevent the crippling effects of osteoporosis.

Up until the age of 35, your body does a pretty good job of balancing the amount of bone that is withdrawn and replaced. But after
the age of 35 most women begin to lose bone faster than they replace
it, at the rate of about one percent of bone mass per year. At this
point, you need to begin working actively to maintain the amount of
bone mass that you have. Although bone loss begins slowly, the rate
increases in the five to eight years around menopause, when women
lose twice as much bone mass per year, for a total loss of 10 to 15

percent of their total bone mass. After this time, bone loss returns to the "normal" rate of one percent per year, but the skeletal structure has been significantly weakened.

The menopausal years are a challenging time for maintaining bone strength because estrogen plays a key role in regulating the ability of the bones to absorb calcium from the blood. Declining estrogen levels, in addition to poor dietary habits and a sedentary lifestyle add up to a significant risk of weakened bones. Osteoporosis can affect all of the bones in the body, but most of the time bone loss is most significant in the spine, hips, and ribs. Most women don't know that they have osteoporosis until they break a bone. Early warning signs of osteoporosis (especially in menopausal women) include chronic low-back pain, loss of height, nocturnal leg cramps, joint pain, and periodontal disease. Often, the first sign is a broken wrist after a minor fall. By the time a woman reaches her sixties, she may have back pain that is caused by bone loss in the spinal vertebrae, and she may have developed the characteristic humped back (dowager's hump) and loss of height that results from compression of the spinal vertebrae. The most serious problems generally show up after the age of 70, when a hip fracture causes serious disability or even death. One of every ten women who suffers a hip fracture will die as a result of complications of the fracture, and most of those who recover will be permanently disabled.

Risk Factors for Osteoporosis

There are clearly defined risk factors for osteoporosis, and many of them are lifestyle factors that you can control. Smoking, excessive alcohol intake, lack of exercise, mineral deficiencies, low body weight caused by excessive dieting or exercise, and a diet high in refined carbohydrates, salt, and excessive protein all contribute to bone loss. Certain diseases, such as irritable bowel syndrome and Crohn's disease, can predispose a woman to osteoporosis because of poor nutrient absorption and an increased loss of calcium caused by chronic diarrhea. Women with diabetes or hypoglycemia are at greater risk because they are more likely to lose calcium when blood-sugar levels are imbalanced. (For information on controlling blood-sugar levels see Chapter 17.) Certain drugs, such as cortisone drugs prescribed for inflammatory diseases and thyroid supplements, if they are in excess of what is needed by the body, can contribute to bone loss. Genetic factors also play a role in osteoporosis: Women who are small-boned and thin, and Caucasian and Asian women have a greater risk than Hispanic or African-American women. If your mother, aunt, or grandmother had osteoporosis, you also have a higher risk. Even if you are at greater risk because of your genetic background, however, your lifestyle choices play the most important role in whether or not you will fall prey to osteoporosis.

If you are at high risk for osteoporosis, it is a good idea to have a screening test to determine your current level of bone density. The best test is DEXA (dual-energy X-ray absorptiometry) which uses a low dose of radiation to measure the vertebrae in the lower back and hip. Urine tests are also available that measure the levels of metabolic compounds that are linked to bone breakdown, which provides information as to the rate of bone loss. These tests are helpful for women with osteoporosis or who are at high risk, because they can help to measure the effectiveness of a treatment program designed to halt bone loss.

Conventional doctors prescribe hormone-replacement therapy (HRT) for decreasing osteoporosis risk. HRT is effective for women who are at high risk for osteoporosis, or for women who already have osteoporosis. But conventional estrogen therapy is not a viable alternative for women who have a history of uterine or breast cancer, heart disease, high blood pressure, liver disease, stroke, diabetes, gallbladder disease, migraine headaches, or blood clots in the veins or lungs. If you have osteoporosis or are at high risk for bone loss, discuss hormone-replacement therapy with your doctor, and explore the possibility of using natural estrogen and progesterone, which appear to have much less risk of unpleasant or dangerous side effects. In any case, dietary changes, exercise, supplements, and herbs can help to prevent and even reverse osteoporosis.

Eating to Build Strong Bones

You might be surprised to learn that calcium is not the only important nutrient for building strong bones. In fact, the United States,

Canada, and the Scandinavian countries are the biggest consumers of dairy products in the world, and yet also suffer the highest rates of osteoporosis. Clearly, simply increasing calcium intake is not the solution to preventing osteoporosis. Despite what milk producers would have you believe, strong bones are not so much related to the amount of calcium in your diet, but are more dependent on whether or not you are absorbing and retaining the calcium you take in. To prevent osteoporosis, you need to eat a diet that contains all of the essential nutrients that make strong bones while avoiding foods that contribute to bone loss, and you need to have good digestion for optimal absorption of nutrients.

There are many factors that contribute to calcium loss and subsequent bone fragility. Dieting is particularly harmful to bones, because low-calorie diets often lack sufficient calcium and other essential nutrients. When not enough minerals are taken in through food, the body draws from the calcium reserves in the bones. Very thin women are at higher risk because fat reserves in the body, particularly in the hips and thighs, help the body to make estrogen, which protects bone mass. Smoking is also detrimental to bone health. Smokers typically go through menopause earlier than non-smokers, which decreases levels of bone-protective estrogen. In addition, smoking suppresses the activity of the parathyroid glands which are responsible for regulating calcium levels.

For calcium to be transported to the bone marrow, it has to be in proper balance with phosphorus. We need some phosphorus for building healthy bones, but the typical daily diet contains much more phosphorus than calcium. For optimal calcium absorption, there should be twice as much calcium as phosphorus in the diet, but most women take in four times as much phosphorus as calcium. Excess phosphorus stimulates the parathyroid glands to secrete a bone-dissolving hormone to maintain the proper calcium-to-phosphorus level. Meats, nuts, seeds, poultry, seafood, dairy products, and whole grains contain large amounts of phosphorus. In addition, phosphorus is added to many processed foods in a variety of forms such as sodium phosphate, phosphoric acid, and potassium phosphate to add flavor or to control the acidity of a product. Carbonated soft drinks are notoriously high in phosphoric acid.

Very low- or very high-protein diets can also cause bone weakness. The amino acids found in proteins are necessary for the body to make bone from calcium. But too much protein (more than about eight ounces per day) can leach calcium from the bones. The digestion of protein produces high levels of nitrogen and sulfur in the blood, creating an acid condition that must be neutralized. Calcium is alkalizing and is used by the body to neutralize these acids, which are then excreted along with calcium in the urine. Women who eat a balanced vegetarian diet tend to have the least incidence of osteoporosis, while women who eat a diet high in meat tend to have the highest rate of bone loss. This doesn't mean that you have to become a vegetarian, but try including more vegetables in your diet, and remove meat from the spotlight. You might also experiment with vegetarian meals that are rich in calcium and other essential nutrients for bone health. See the recipes in Appendix I for a variety of delicious vegetarian meals based on tofu, tempeh, and legumes.

Other dietary factors that contribute to bone loss include caffeine, alcohol, and excessive salt and sugar. Caffeine, found in coffee, black tea, chocolate, caffeinated soft drinks, and some over-the-counter medications, has diuretic properties (it increases urination) and doubles the rate of calcium that is lost in the urine. Coffee has some additional negative effects, because the acids that it contains are neutralized by calcium that is drawn from the bones. Too much salt and sugar also cause the kidneys to excrete calcium in the urine, and excess alcohol (more than about three drinks per week) has a suppressive effect on hormonal function, which exacerbates bone loss.

A whole-foods, nutrient-rich diet is essential for preventing and treating osteoporosis. Dairy foods are touted as the best way to strengthen bones, and it is true that they are rich sources of calcium. However, many women have difficulty digesting dairy products, and dairy is also high in phosphorus, which can interfere with calcium absorption. There are many other foods that are excellent sources of calcium without the drawbacks of dairy foods. Dark-green leafy vegetables, broccoli, tofu, sesame seeds, almonds, and canned salmon and sardines eaten with the bones are just a few calcium-rich nondairy foods. Some dairy products are easier to digest than others, especially those that are fermented, such as yogurt. If you digest dairy easily, by all means include it as a good source of calcium. But whether or not dairy foods agree with you, broaden your diet to include a wide variety of calcium-rich foods that offer you a wide range of essential bone-building nutrients in addition to calcium.

CALCIUM-RICH FOODS

Collard greens, 1 cup cooked	350 mg
Sardines, 4 ounces	450 mg
Yogurt, 8 ounces	300 mg
Kale, 1 cup cooked	200 mg
Mustard greens, 1 cup cooked	190 mg
Salmon, canned, 3 ounces	170 mg
Dandelion greens, 1 cup cooked	150 mg
Tofu, 4 ounces	150 mg
Almonds, 1/2 cup	150 mg
Broccoli, 1 cup cooked	145 mg
Corn tortillas, 2	120 mg
Sesame seeds, 1 tablespoon	90 mg

Although calcium is not the only nutrient necessary for bone health, it is one of the most essential, and calcium supplements play an important role in preventing and treating osteoporosis. To ensure bone health, take 1,000 to 1,500 milligrams of calcium daily. If you eat plenty of calcium-rich foods every day, the lower dosage is sufficient. The best form of supplemental calcium is calcium citrate, which is easily absorbed. Other good forms are aspartate, lactate, gluconate, and malate, but avoid supplements made from bone meal, oyster shell, and dolomite. Not only are they poorly broken down and absorbed by the body, but they are likely to be contaminated with lead, a toxic metal that accumulates in the body. Calcium antacids are often promoted as calcium supplements, but because they alkalize stomach acids, they inhibit calcium absorption and increase the risk of kidney stones. When taking calcium supplements, it's best to divide the amount into two doses daily, because your digestive tract can absorb only a certain amount of calcium at one time. Take one dose at night before bedtime, when most bone loss occurs.

Little-Known Nutrients for Bone Health

So much emphasis is given to calcium for preventing osteoporosis that other essential nutrients are often overlooked. Not only calcium, but vitamin D, vitamin K, and the minerals magnesium, manganese, boron, zinc, and copper are necessary for healthy bones. Eating a varied diet is the best way to get most of these nutrients, as well as taking a high-potency vitamin-and-mineral supplement for added insurance. Dark-green leafy vegetables such as romaine, kale, mustard greens, collard greens, parsley, and broccoli are packed with nutrients that keep bones healthy. Not only are they high in calcium and the trace mineral boron, but they are also rich sources of vitamin K, a little-known nutrient that is critical for regulating blood-calcium levels and for bone formation. About half of the vitamin K that you need is made by beneficial bacteria in the intestinal tract. To encourage a healthy population of friendly intestinal flora, eat yogurt that contains live acidophilus cultures. You can also take *Lactobacillus acidophilus* supplements that contain at least one billion live organisms daily before breakfast for one month or longer.

Vitamin D helps the gastrointestinal tract absorb calcium and ensures that there is enough calcium in the blood for adequate bone formation. Often referred to as the "sunshine vitamin," vitamin D is produced by your body from sunlight. When the sun's rays come into contact with your skin, a cholesterol compound in the skin is transformed into vitamin D. It only takes about 15 minutes of sun exposure in the midmorning or late afternoon three days a week to fulfill your requirement, but glass, clothing, and smog all block the ultraviolet rays that help your body create vitamin D. Eggs, butter, and fortified milk also contain vitamin D. In excess, vitamin D can contribute to heart disease, kidney damage, and tissue calcification. The best way to obtain this essential vitamin is through moderate exposure to sunshine, which has been shown to be better than supplements for promoting calcium absorption and bone strength. However, many women with osteoporosis may have difficulties with making vitamin D. Therefore, many experts recommend taking supplements of up to 400 units of vitamin D daily.

Magnesium is also essential for building strong bones and helps to prevent calcium from being excreted by the body. Although magnesium is found in many foods, such as nuts, seeds, legumes, whole grains, seafood, and leafy greens, many women do not get enough of this critical nutrient. In addition to low intake of magnesium-rich foods, this important mineral is depleted by emotional and physical stress, exercise, and alcohol. To ensure an adequate intake of magnesium, eat foods rich in magnesium daily and take 400 to 600 milligrams daily of magnesium, preferably in the form of magnesium citrate, aspartate, gluconate, or lactate, all easily absorbable forms of the mineral.

Including foods that are good sources of phytoestrogens such as tofu, tempeh, and flaxseeds can help to prevent bone loss by increasing levels of estrogen and helping to balance hormone levels. For optimal protection against bone loss, you need to eat significant amounts of these foods on a daily basis. Nutritionists estimate that one unit of estrogen is roughly equivalent to one tablespoon of flaxseeds, one cup of soymilk, four ounces of tofu or tempeh, or one-third cup of soybeans or soyflour. To protect against osteoporosis, you need to eat about three servings of phytoestrogen-rich foods every day. See Appendix I for ideas for including these foods in your diet.

Build Bone Strength with Exercise

While optimal nutrition is critical for bone health, regular exercise is equally essential. The old adage "use it or lose it" is particularly appropriate as a mandate for maintaining strong bones. A sedentary life weakens bones—even one week of bedrest causes loss of bone density. On the other hand, bones respond to physical exertion by becoming thicker and stronger. When bones are subjected to the stress of weight-bearing exercise, a mild electrical-energy charge is generated that stimulates calcium to be deposited in the bones. Weight-bearing exercises such as brisk walking, jogging, tennis, skiing, and dancing are best for building bone. Although swimming can benefit your cardiovascular system, it doesn't increase bone strength because the buoyancy of the water prevents you from putting stress on your bones. To build bone, you must be working against gravity, which creates the energy charge that stimulates bone to grow. Upper-body exercises, such as weight lifting and heavy gardening, are as important as lower-body exercises for strengthening bone. In general, plan for a minimum of three hours per week of weight-bearing exercise to protect bone health.

As you age, regular exercise becomes more critical than ever not only for maintaining bone mass, but also for improving balance and coordination. Many older people develop a shuffling gait and a lack of coordination that is caused by weak muscles and a general decline in fitness. They frequently curtail their activities because they are afraid of falling, which causes them to become even weaker and more accident prone. The stronger you are and the more confident you feel in your body, the less likely you are to suffer an accident such as a fall, which is the most common cause of broken bones. If you haven't already done so, begin a regular exercise program now that will enable you to remain active and vital throughout your life. Even if you already have osteoporosis, weight-bearing exercise can help to slow down the rate of bone loss and may even help to build new bone. Note that while frequent, regular exercise is excellent for your bones and your overall health, overdoing it (such as training for marathons) can be counterproductive, because it can diminish estrogen levels and also increase the possibility of bone fractures.

Most women find it easier to undertake a program of weight-bearing exercise that benefits the lower body and tend to neglect upper-body strength, which is equally important for bone health. As a result, many find themselves with muscles so weak that they cannot comfortably carry a heavy package or unscrew a tight jar lid. Although modern life offers little in the way of daily activities to strengthen the upper body, a simple strengthening routine performed with hand-held weights two or three times a week for 20 to 30 minutes will build strength and keep bones strong. If you prefer, you can work out at a gym using weight-training machines. A side benefit of strengthening exercises is that they work quickly to improve your appearance by firming and shaping your muscles.

An ideal weight-training program consists of eight to ten exercises that work all of the major muscle groups—arms, shoulders, abdominals, buttocks, and legs. Take a class or schedule a few sessions with a professional exercise trainer who can show you how to perform weight-lifting exercises correctly. Lift enough weight so that your muscles are fatigued after eight to ten repetitions. The goal is to tire your muscles so that they are stimulated to become stronger (which will in turn strengthen your bones), but at no time should you feel pain. You may need to start with light weights, even one or two pounds. When the exercise becomes easy, increase the weight so that you are continuing to gain strength. Always lift weights slowly and smoothly, and never make jerky or fast movements that can injure your joints. Be sure to breathe while you are exercising, and exhale when you are performing the most difficult part of the exercise. Warm up before weight training with at least five minutes of aerobic exercise, and cool down afterwards with ten minutes of stretching to relax the muscles that you have just worked. Give yourself one full day or more between weight-training sessions to allow your muscles time to recover.

Herbs for Healthy Bones

Although herbs alone cannot prevent or reverse osteoporosis, they are a valuable addition to building and maintaining bone health. Herbs that are rich in phytoestrogens, such as *dong quai* and *black cohosh,* help to balance hormones and provide estrogenic support. Take the *Hormone-Balancing Tonic* on page 86 daily. Herbs that support the functioning of the endocrine glands, such as *Siberian ginseng* and *American ginseng,* also help to keep bones strong. After the age of 40, digestive function is often less than optimal, and the stomach and digestive organs may not produce enough stomach acids and enzymes for the breakdown and assimilation of the nutrients that are essential for bone health. To ensure optimal assimilation of nutrients, follow the suggestions in Chapter 20 for improving digestive function, and take the *Herbal Digestive Tonic* on page 197 before meals to aid digestion.

Many herbs are rich sources of bone-building nutrients, especially trace minerals and vitamin K. Eat *dandelion greens, watercress,* and *parsley* often. Dandelion greens are one of the most nutritious leafy green vegetables—they have more calcium and iron than spinach and also contain magnesium, phosphorus, zinc, and other trace minerals. They have a hearty, mildly bitter flavor similar to endive and are delicious sauteed, steamed, or in salads. You probably have dandelion greens growing in your backyard, and some groceries carry fresh dandelion greens. Harvest dandelion greens in the early spring, before the flowers appear, and again in the late fall after a frost. If you harvest dandelion from the wild, make sure that you know what you are harvesting and only gather plants that have not been sprayed with chemicals. See the resource section on page 338 for suggestions for field guides for information on harvesting wild plants. A tea made from fresh or dried dandelion greens stimulates digestive juices and helps to improve the assimilation of nutrients. Pour one cup of boiling water over one to two teaspoons of dried dandelion leaf, cover, and steep for ten minutes. Strain and drink 15 minutes before meals.

Nettle *(Urtica dioica)* contains a wide variety of nutrients, including calcium, magnesium, vitamin K, and trace minerals, as well as easily absorbable amino acids. The dried herb is readily available and makes a good-tasting tea, and if you have fresh nettle growing nearby, it makes a wonderful vegetable dish when sautéed. To make nettle tea, pour one cup of boiling water over two teaspoons of dried nettle. Cover, and steep for ten minutes. Strain, and drink three cups daily.

Horsetail *(Equisetum arvense)* is high in calcium and other trace minerals including silica, which traditionally is used to stimulate bone regeneration. Add horsetail to other mineral-rich herbs to help to strengthen bones. The following tea contains a variety of herbs that are good sources of the minerals that help to build healthy bones.

Bone Strengthening Tea

4 tablespoons nettle
1 tablespoon horsetail
1 tablespoon red clover blossoms
3 cups water

Pour boiling water over herbs, cover, and steep 1 hour or longer. Strain, pressing the herbs to remove as much liquid as possible. Drink 3 cups daily.

Chapter 22

How to Keep Your Heart Healthy

We have a tendency in this country to think of heart disease as something that happens to men, and until fairly recently, little attention has been paid to the health of women's hearts. It's true that before menopause, women are unlikely to suffer from cardiovascular disease because of the protective effects of estrogen. After menopause, however, we quickly catch up to men and are even slightly *more* likely to be stricken with heart disease. Overall, cardiovascular disease is the leading cause of death for American women, affecting one out of every three women over the age of 65. The most common cardiovascular diseases are heart attack and stroke, which often strike without prior warning, and if they don't kill, frequently cause serious physical and mental impairment that greatly interfere with the quality of life.

But you don't have to fall victim to cardiovascular disease. The major contributing factors to both heart attacks and strokes are atherosclerosis, which is a thickening and hardening of the arteries, and high blood pressure. Both of these conditions are almost entirely within your control. Your doctor may try to convince you to take estrogen to prevent cardiovascular disease, but there are significant side effects associated with hormone therapy, including an increased risk of life-threatening blood clots and some types of stroke. Because cardiovascular disease is largely a disease of lifestyle, natural methods of healing that include diet, exercise, and herbal treatments are extremely effective. Prevention is always best, but even if you have been diagnosed with atherosclerosis or high blood pressure, natural treatments can help to *reverse* the disease.

Six Keys for Cardiovascular Health

Eat a Nutrient-Dense Diet

Populations with a low incidence of cardiovascular disease eat diets that are rich in vegetables, grains, legumes, and fish. Such diets provide a wealth of protective nutrients such as antioxidants, essential fatty acids, minerals, and fiber that keep cholesterol levels balanced, arteries clean and flexible, and blood pressure low. Eating a nutrient-dense diet provides more protection for your cardiovascular system than simply slashing fat and cholesterol from your diet, which can actually do more harm than good. Follow the recommendations for a health-enhancing diet in Chapter 26, along with the specific recommendations in this chapter and Chapters 23 and 24 for preventing atherosclerosis and high blood pressure if these conditions apply to you.

Saturate Your Cells with Antioxidants

Antioxidants are critical for keeping your cardiovascular system healthy. They prevent damage to your heart and arteries caused by free radicals, mutant molecules that are generated by a variety of factors including exposure to environmental toxins, chemicals in food and water, unhealthful fats and processed foods, cigarette smoke, emotional stress, overwork, and insufficient sleep. Free radicals are also a normal by-product of metabolic processes. Your body has a number of built-in antioxidant mechanisms that help to neutralize free radicals and repair the damage they cause. Problems arise when large numbers of free radicals overwhelm your body's capacity to stabilize them, which leads to escalating tissue damage, degenerative disease, and aging. Boosting your intake of concentrated antioxidants such as fresh fruits and vegetables, green tea, beta-carotene and other carotenoids, vitamin C, vitamin E, grapeseed extract, and selenium floods your body with protective nutrients that prevent cell damage.

Avoid Exposure to Toxins

Every time you are exposed to toxins such as tobacco, pesticides, herbicides, solvents, household and gardening chemicals, and over-the-counter and prescription drugs, free radicals are generated in your body that increase your risk of cardiovascular disease. To avoid exposure to toxins, buy organic foods, use filtered water, avoid tobacco smoke (including secondhand smoke), use herbs and other natural remedies instead of pharmaceutical drugs, and choose natural alternatives to household and gardening chemicals that are not harmful to you or the environment.

Exercise Regularly

Regular moderate exercise is essential for cardiovascular health. Your heart is a muscle, and it becomes a stronger and more efficient pump with exercise. Regular exercise also improves your circulation, reduces harmful cholesterol, lowers your blood pressure, and provides a healthful avenue for easing the emotional tension that contributes to cardiovascular disease. Aerobic exercise doesn't have to be uncomfortably strenuous to be beneficial. Any exercise that gets you breathing more deeply and slightly increases your heart rate is strengthening for your cardiovascular system. The most important guideline is to exercise frequently—plan for at least 30 minutes five days a week.

Learn to Manage Stress

Emotional tension plays a critical role in the development of cardiovascular disease. When you are emotionally stressed, hormones such as adrenaline are released into your bloodstream that increase your heart rate and raise your blood pressure. Chronic stress weakens your heart and arteries, raises levels of unhealthful cholesterol, increases free radical destruction, and causes your blood pressure to remain abnormally high. Deep breathing exercises, yoga, and meditation are excellent for helping to relax your body and your mind, and practicing these techniques regularly will help to keep your heart and circulatory system healthy and strong.

Take Herbal Cardiovascular Tonics

For centuries in Europe, China, and India, people have used herbs as rejuvenative tonics to keep their hearts and arteries strong and healthy. Herbs provide concentrated nutrients and healing compounds that prevent cardiovascular disease and help to relieve atherosclerosis and high blood pressure. When taken on a regular basis, cardiovascular tonics such as *garlic, hawthorne,* and *ginkgo* help to maintain healthy cholesterol levels, keep arteries flexible, strengthen heart function, improve circulation, and prevent free-radical damage.

Two Little-Known Risk Factors for Heart Disease

Because cholesterol has been tagged as the primary culprit in cardiovascular disease, other factors that are equally important are frequently overlooked. Two compounds found in the blood called homocysteine and fibrinogen wreak havoc with arteries and may be even more dangerous than cholesterol. Homocysteine is a by-product of the metabolism of the amino acid methionine, and it can become oxidized just as LDL cholesterol does. When it oxidizes, it releases a lethal free radical called superoxide, which is thought to be even more destructive to your arteries than oxidized cholesterol. If you are healthy, homocysteine is neutralized by your body into harmless compounds before it can cause damage, but if you are deficient in B-complex vitamins (specifically folic acid, vitamin B-6, or vitamin B-12) homocysteine levels can increase in your blood to dangerous levels. High levels of homocysteine directly damage the arteries by attacking blood-vessel walls, promoting the buildup of fatty plaque, and increasing dangerous blood clotting that can cause heart attacks and strokes.

Fibrinogen is a protein in blood that is essential for blood clotting. It makes blood sticky, which is a lifesaving function if your body needs to staunch bleeding, but having too much fibrinogen makes your blood overly sticky, causing it to clump together and creating life-threatening blood clots. High levels of fibrinogen are directly related to coronary-artery disease, high blood pressure, heart attacks, and strokes. Factors that increase fibrinogen are high levels of LDL cholesterol, smoking, obesity, high blood-sugar levels, emotional stress, and supplemental estrogen in hormone-replacement therapy and birth-control pills. To keep fibrinogen levels in a healthy range, exercise regularly and eat a diet rich in nutrients that decrease the stickiness of blood platelets such as garlic, the essential fatty acids found in cold-water fish, and the protective antioxidants found in fresh vegetables and fruits.

Eating for a Healthy Heart

What you eat on a daily basis is a powerful factor in the health of your cardiovascular system. Through the foods you choose to eat (and the foods you avoid) you can increase your levels of protective HDL cholesterol while lowering your levels of harmful oxidized LDL cholesterol, homocysteine, and fibrinogen. Measurable changes show up quickly in your blood, usually within a few weeks.

Knowing how much and what kind of fats to eat has been an area of much controversy, with some experts recommending an extremely low-fat diet (less than 10 percent) with no animal foods, and some recommending eating as much fat as you want, including saturated fats. The healthiest approach, as with many things in life, is probably somewhere in between. While an extremely low-fat diet has been proven to decrease cholesterol levels, such a drastic approach is difficult or impossible for most people to live with and can cause other health problems, such as skin dryness, hair loss, depression, and lowered immunity. Fat is not an optional nutrient—it is an essential building block for health, just as important as protein and carbohydrates. The *right* kinds of fats have a protective effect, and it is vitally important that you pay attention to the types

of fats you eat. You can't eat fried foods, red meats, polyunsaturated oils, margarine, and baked goods made with hydrogenated oils
and expect to stay healthy. But you can, and should, eat plenty of
heart-healthy fats in the form of cold-water fish, raw nuts and seeds,
avocados, and olive oil.

In general, it's a good idea to keep your fat intake to no more
than 30 percent of your total daily calories. Saturated fats (found primarily in animal foods and in some vegetable fats such as palm-ker-
nel oil and coconut oil) should add up to no more than 10 percent
of your daily calories or even less. Don't ever eat hydrogenated fats,
which have undergone a chemical process that makes them solid at
room temperature and creates toxic and cell-damaging compounds
called transfatty acids. These dangerous fats are found in margarine,
vegetable shortening, and many processed and packaged foods that
are made with hydrogenated or partially hydrogenated oils. Polyunsaturated oils such as safflower, corn, and sunflower, all of which
have been promoted as being healthful for your heart, are not. They
quickly turn rancid, many times even while on the store shelves,
and once in your body create free radicals that transform LDL
cholesterol into its harmful oxidized form.

Healthful fats for your cardiovascular system include those rich
in monounsaturated fats, which are stable and slow to oxidize in
your kitchen or in your body. Cultures that eat diets rich in monounsaturated fats—such as the Mediterranean cultures—have a significantly lower incidence of cardiovascular disease. Olive oil and
avocados are rich in monounsaturated fats, as are walnuts and
almonds. Olive oil is also rich in oleic acid, which makes cholesterol
less susceptible to free-radical damage. Olive oil offers many benefits for the cardiovascular system—it increases HDL cholesterol, lowers LDL cholesterol, and helps to make the capillary walls more
flexible and stronger. Be sure to buy extra-virgin olive oil, which is
the purest form and has not been diluted with polyunsaturated oils.
Although avocados and raw nuts are high in fat they help to
decrease total cholesterol levels and reduce LDL cholesterol without
lowering levels of HDL. Buy fresh, raw nuts and seeds, preferably
from a store that keeps them refrigerated, and store them in the
refrigerator at home to keep them fresh.

The omega-3 fatty acids found in cold-water fish are especially
important for cardiovascular health. They help to decrease cholesterol
and block the dangerous oxidation of LDL cholesterol, reduce triglyc-

erides, and prevent excessive blood-platelet stickiness, which inhibits the formation of dangerous blood clots. To protect your heart and arteries, eat salmon, sardines, albacore tuna, halibut, and mackerel three to four times a week. Fish-oil supplements are sometimes recommended for providing the healthful oils found in fish, but they are often rancid and may do more harm than good. They are *not* a healthful substitute for eating fresh fish. If you are a vegetarian and opposed to eating fish, you can take one tablespoon per day of flaxseed oil, which is the richest vegetable source of omega-3 fatty acids.

Eating plenty of foods rich in soluble fibers such as oats, barley, and cooked dried beans helps to reduce cholesterol by binding to it in the intestinal tract and excreting it from the body. Another type of important cholesterol-lowering fiber called pectin is found in apples, carrots, and the inner white rind of citrus fruits. If you want to increase your intake of soluble fiber, eat a bowl of oatmeal several days a week for breakfast, a marinated bean salad or a bean soup for lunch a few days a week, and a carrot and apple for snacks every day. When you eat citrus fruits, make it a point to eat a bit of the white inner peel. To increase your fiber intake even more, you can take a fiber supplement that contains both psyllium seed and pectin. Take one teaspoon two to three times a day with a full glass of water.

Although the primary dietary strategy for preventing cardiovascular disease is focused on fat and cholesterol, limiting your intake of sugar is equally important. High-sugar foods raise levels of triglycerides, cholesterol, and insulin and increase the stickiness of blood platelets. Sugar in all forms—honey, molasses, highly concentrated fruit sweeteners, and maple syrup—raises blood-sugar levels and takes a toll on the cardiovascular system. Read the labels on low-fat packaged cookies, sorbets, and other snacks; they are often loaded with a variety of sugars, which makes them harmful, not healthful choices. You can keep your sugar intake to a minimum by substituting fresh fruits for sugary snacks and making sweet and rich desserts an occasional treat instead of a daily habit.

Supplements for Cardiovascular Health

In addition to eating a varied whole-foods diet rich in heart-protecting nutrients, taking a variety of supplements provides extra health insurance for your cardiovascular system.

- The B-complex vitamins folic acid, B-6, and B-12 help to prevent the build-up of artery-damaging homocysteine in the blood. For most women, taking a high-complex B supplement that provides 400 micrograms of folic acid, 50 milligrams of B-6, and 400 micrograms of B-12 is sufficient for keeping homocysteine levels down. If you have high levels of homocysteine, you may need higher amounts of these B-vitamins. Work with your health care practitioner to determine the optimum dosage.

- Vitamin E provides antioxidant protection and prevents the oxidation of LDL cholesterol. It also inhibits the formation of arterial plaque and reduces the risk of dangerous blood clots. Take 400 to 800 units of vitamin E in the form of d-alpha tocopherol daily.

- Vitamin C provides antioxidant protection, supports the action of vitamin E, and prevents the oxidation of LDL cholesterol. It also helps to strengthen the blood vessels. Take 1,000 to 2,000 milligrams daily in divided doses two to three times a day.

- Coenzyme Q-10 is an enzyme that is vital for the production of energy within the cells and is found in especially high concentrations in the heart. CoQ-10 is fat soluble, and is able to enter the molecules of LDL cholesterol to prevent oxidation. It also helps to strengthen the heart and decrease blood pressure. Take CoQ-10 in gel capsules with a meal that contains fat to aid in absorption. As a protective dose, take 30 to 60 milligrams once a day. If you have cardiovascular disease, take up to 240 milligrams a day divided into two equal doses.

- Magnesium helps to dilate the coronary arteries, enhances energy production in the heart, improves blood flow to the heart, increases levels of beneficial HDL cholesterol, prevents blood platelets from clumping together, and stabilizes heart rhythm. Good sources of magnesium include legumes, nuts, seeds, whole grains, and tofu. In addition to eating foods rich in magnesium, take 400 to 600 milligrams of magnesium daily in the form of magnesium citrate, asparate, gluconate, or lactate, all forms that are easily absorbed.

- Grapeseed extract is a rich source of natural compounds called proanthocyanidins, powerful antioxidants that are at least 20 times more potent than vitamin C or E. These compounds inhibit the oxidation of LDL cholesterol, prevent damage to arteries, strengthen the blood-vessel walls, improve circulation, and prevent the clumping of blood platelets. Take 50 milligrams daily as a preventive dose and 150 milligrams daily if you have high cholesterol or heart disease.

- Niacin in large doses is extremely effective at lowering total cholesterol and LDL levels while raising levels of beneficial HDL. Taking large amounts of niacin can cause a harmless flushing of the chest and face. To prevent this reaction, take inositol hexanicotinate, and start with a low dose of 50 milligrams three times a day, gradually increasing to 400 milligrams two to three times a day. Avoid sustained-release niacin, which can cause liver toxicity. If you have diabetes, take large amounts of niacin only under the supervision of your doctor, because it can interfere with blood-sugar levels.

  If you want to use niacin therapeutically, your cholesterol and liver enzyme levels should be monitored by your doctor. You will usually see positive results within two months, although very high cholesterol levels (above 300 mg/dl) may take up to six months or even one year to respond sufficiently. When your cholesterol levels fall below 200 mg/dl, gradually taper off the niacin and check your cholesterol levels after two months. If your cholesterol increases, resume taking the niacin until your cholesterol has stabilized below 200 mg/dl.

- If you are postmenopausal, avoid excess iron, including iron-fortified foods and multivitamin supplements containing iron. Iron easily accumulates in the blood, where it promotes free radicals that change cholesterol into the oxidized form that attacks arteries.

The Best Herbal Tonics for Your Heart

Herbs cannot take the place of a healthful diet, exercise, and stress management, but they are an important component of a program for optimal cardiovascular health. The following herbs can be used on a daily basis to keep your heart and circulatory system in top condition and are excellent as part of a treatment program for atherosclerosis and hypertension and other cardiovascular conditions such as arrhythmias, angina, and congestive heart failure. These herbs have a long history of safe use and are most effective when taken on a long-term basis. *If you have a serious cardiovascular condition, work with a professional herbalist or a physician skilled in herbal medicine to design a program that will be most helpful for you.*

Garlic *(Allium sativum)* is a powerful cardiovascular tonic in a small pungent package. The sulfur compounds that give garlic its characteristic odor are responsible for the health benefits of the herb. It lowers harmful LDL cholesterol and triglycerides and increases beneficial HDL cholesterol, reduces dangerous clotting by inhibiting blood-platelet clumping, lowers blood pressure, and prevents the oxidation of fat and cholesterol that causes artery damage. Raw garlic has more potent properties than cooked, but either one is helpful. There's no need to buy garlic supplements. It takes only one to two cloves of garlic per day to protect your cardiovascular system. If you absolutely cannot tolerate fresh garlic, take a standardized extract that provides a daily dose of at least ten milligrams of alliin, which is equal to approximately one clove of fresh garlic.

Ginkgo *(Ginkgo biloba)* is an ancient tree whose leaves have been used in herbal medicine for more than 4,000 years in China. Rich in antioxidant compounds, ginkgo improves circulation and blood flow to the heart, strengthens blood vessels, and reduces the risk of blood clots that can cause heart attacks and strokes. Ginkgo also improves blood flow to the extremities, which is helpful for relieving intermittent claudication, a condition caused by atherosclerosis where blood flow to the legs is impaired. Take an extract of ginkgo standardized to contain 24 percent ginkgo heterosides, 40 milligrams three times a day.

Hawthorne *(Crataegus oxycantha)* has been used for centuries in Europe as a heart-strengthening tonic and is appropriate for treating virtually every type of cardiovascular disorder. The flowers, leaves, and fruit of the hawthorne tree or shrub contain potent antioxidant compounds called flavonoids that have a special affinity for the heart and arteries. These beneficial compounds help to increase blood flow to the heart, dilate the arteries, strengthen and steady the heartbeat, and reduce blood pressure. Hawthorne also lowers harmful LDL cholesterol and triglycerides, inhibits cholesterol from attaching to artery walls, and helps to dissolve existing fatty plaque. Because hawthorne helps to regulate the heartbeat, it can alleviate heart rhythm disturbances, and by improving blood flow to the heart, it helps to relieve angina. Mild to moderate cases of congestive heart failure may be eased by hawthorne. As a preventive tonic, drink hawthorne as a tea. Pour one cup of boiling water over two teaspoons of dried berries, leaves, and flowers, cover, and steep for 15 minutes. Strain and drink two cups per day. Hawthorne makes a pleasant-tasting, slightly sweet tea. If you have cardiovascular disease, take one teaspoon of hawthorne extract three times per day, or 200 milligrams of a standardized extract three times per day.

Chapter 23

Avoid Developing Atherosclerosis

Commonly known as hardening of the arteries, atherosclerosis often causes no symptoms until the arteries are narrowed so severely that a heart attack or stroke occurs. Atherosclerosis is almost entirely a disease of lifestyle and is caused by the buildup of fatty plaque in the arteries that is composed of cholesterol, other fats, and cellular debris. Risk factors for coronary-artery disease include cigarette smoking, high blood pressure, high cholesterol levels (especially high levels of LDL cholesterol), high triglyceride levels, low levels of HDL cholesterol, diabetes, obesity, a high-fat or high-sugar diet, emotional stress, a sedentary lifestyle, and a family history of the disease. Except for the genetic connection, all other factors are within your control, and while a family history of the disease may predispose you to developing atherosclerosis, lifestyle factors are far more important.

Cholesterol-lowering drugs are often prescribed to lower blood-cholesterol levels, but have dangerous side effects, including an increased incidence of cancer and severe emotional disturbances such as depression and anxiety. Aspirin is frequently recommended for preventing heart attacks and strokes because it thins the blood and inhibits the formation of dangerous blood clots. But aspirin is not a harmless substance—taking it long term can cause bleeding in the digestive tract and liver toxicity, and it can suppress immune function. Common surgeries for heart disease include angioplasty, where a catheter is inserted into an artery and a tiny balloon is inflated to compress the fatty plaque and open up the artery, but it is not a cure for the disease. Artery blockage tends to recur, often within a period of months. Bypass surgery is also frequently performed, where a vein is taken from the leg and grafted onto the narrowed coronary artery to bypass the one that is clogged, but again, blockage tends to recur. Lifestyle changes are much safer and more effective than either cholesterol-lowering drugs or aspirin and are certainly an infinitely better choice than surgery. The only side effects to lifestyle changes are positive, health-enhancing ones.

The Truth About Cholesterol

You might be surprised to learn that cholesterol is not the villain that it is made out to be in the disease of atherosclerosis. High cholesterol levels are associated with clogged arteries, but simply eating a low-fat, low-cholesterol diet is not the answer. While cholesterol has been targeted as the major cause of clogged arteries, the picture is far more complex, with other factors such as homocysteine, fibrinogen, and free radicals playing destructive roles in initiating the disease.

It's important to look at the total cholesterol picture, because there are many factors to consider. Cholesterol is a waxy, yellow fat that is found in every cell of your body. While you may think of it as a harmful substance, it's actually vital to your health. Cholesterol is necessary for the production of hormones, vitamin D, bile, and cell membranes. Even if you eat no cholesterol whatsoever, your body will manufacture it, because it is necessary for your well-being. Cholesterol becomes a problem only when you are lacking dietary nutrients that are essential for it to be metabolized correctly, or when a sedentary lifestyle or poor liver function cause it to build up to unhealthy levels in your bloodstream and arteries.

Cholesterol is transported through your blood on molecules called lipoproteins. Low-density lipoproteins (LDL) carry cholesterol and triglycerides from your liver to your cells, and high-density lipoproteins (HDL) return the same fats to your liver to be metabolized and excreted. While high levels of LDL cholesterol are linked to an increased risk of atherosclerosis, high levels of HDL cholesterol are associated with a low risk of artery disease. If you have low levels of protective HDL cholesterol, you have an increased risk of coronary artery disease even if your total cholesterol count is within the normal range. High levels of trigylcerides, another blood fat, also increase the risk of atherosclerosis. To prevent coronary-artery disease, heart attacks, and strokes, you need to lower your blood levels of LDL cholesterol and triglycerides and increase your blood level of protective HDL cholesterol. For most women, these changes can happen within weeks or months simply by making dietary and lifestyle changes.

Here are the facts to help you decipher the meaning of your cholesterol reading: Your total cholesterol levels should be less than 200 mg/dl, your LDL no higher than 130 (preferably closer to 100), your triglycerides less than 150 mg/dl, and your HDL greater than 35. The risk of heart disease increases dramatically with cholesterol readings over 200, and even though this is considered a normal rating, it is probably healthier to strive for a lower cholesterol reading of somewhere around 160. You don't want to go too low, however, because extremely low cholesterol levels (below 150) are associated with an increased risk of other diseases such as cancer and depression.

Even more important than the individual numbers in your cholesterol reading is the ratio of your HDL cholesterol to your total cholesterol, and also the ratio of LDL to HDL in your blood. This indicates whether cholesterol is being adequately broken down by your liver and excreted from your body, or whether it is being deposited in your arteries. The ideal ratio of HDL to total cholesterol is below 3.5, with 3.5 to 4.5 considered average, and above 4.5 a higher-than-average risk. The ratio of LDL to HDL should be no higher than 2.5. You can reduce your risk of heart disease by taking steps to lower your LDL cholesterol and trigylcerides and to raise your HDL cholesterol, but there are other factors that contribute to the development of atherosclerosis that are equally and possibly even more important to consider.

When Cholesterol Becomes a Problem

The process of atherosclerosis begins when the cells that line the inside of the artery are damaged by free radicals, which can be generated by environmental or internal toxins, stress, or viruses. As a protective measure, the body repairs the damage with fatty plaque to strengthen the artery where it has been weakened and to prevent it from possibly rupturing. However, this narrows the artery and makes it more susceptible to blockage from blood clots. Free radicals also make blood platelets more sticky, which increases the risk of blood clots, and affect LDL cholesterol, transforming it into a particularly nasty substance called oxidized cholesterol. This type of LDL cholesterol damages artery walls and more easily builds up into arterial plaque that clogs arteries. Free radicals are continually being created in your body, and your body is constantly striving to neutralize them to prevent damage from accumulating. The best approach you can take to prevent free-radical damage is to live a healthful lifestyle, limit your exposure to toxins, and keep your cells saturated with antioxidant nutrients from foods, supplements, and herbs.

How to Shield Your Arteries from Free Radicals

You can take steps today to protect your arteries from free-radical damage by supporting your body's production of antioxidant compounds and by increasing your intake of these cell-protecting nutrients. One of the most powerful antioxidants working to protect you is glutathione, a compound made by your body. Glutathione helps to detoxify harmful oxidized fats in the intestinal tract, preventing them from entering the bloodstream and causing free-radical damage. Levels of glutathione tend to decrease with age, and production is also impaired by dietary and environmental toxins that stress the liver. You can increase your levels of glutathione by eating lots of fresh fruits and vegetables. Some of the richest sources include avocados, asparagus, grapefruit, watermelon, and strawberries. You can also boost your body's production of glutathione by eating cruciferous vegetables such as cabbage, cauliflower, and broccoli and consuming foods high in the amino acid cysteine, such as onions, garlic, and yogurt. Vitamin C also helps to stimulate the production of glutathione, as does the antioxidant mineral selenium.

Centering your diet around a variety of fresh vegetables and fruits provides a wealth of protective nutrients that both prevent free-radical damage and help to cleanse your arteries. Fresh vegetables and fruits contain compounds called phytosterols, which help to remove cholesterol from your bloodstream. Foods that are especially rich in these beneficial cleansing nutrients include asparagus, cauliflower, spinach, onions, strawberries, apricots, celery, tomatoes, lettuce, cucumbers, and figs. Another way to boost your intake of antioxidants is to drink green tea, which contains potent protective compounds called polyphenols that help to lower cholesterol and trigylcerides, block the oxidation of LDL cholesterol, and prevent the dangerous clumping of blood platelets. Drink three cups a day of green tea—it makes an excellent substitute for coffee or black tea and has mild energizing properties. In moderate amounts, red wine also appears to have a beneficial effect on the cardiovascular system. Like green tea, red wine contains polyphenols that help to prevent the oxidation of LDL cholesterol. If you enjoy an occasional glass of wine, choose organic red wine, and limit your intake to one glass a few times a week. You can also obtain the same protective compounds from purple grapes and purple grape juice.

Two Ayurvedic Herbs for Healthy Arteries

Some of the most important herbs for maintaining healthy arteries are *hawthorne, garlic,* and *ginkgo,* which were discussed on page 224 as tonics for the cardiovascular system. In addition, the following herbs from the Ayurvedic herbal tradition are highly beneficial for treating elevated cholesterol levels and atherosclerosis.

Turmeric *(Curcuma longa)* is best known as a culinary spice used in Indian curries, and it is also the ingredient that gives mustard its bright yellow color. It has powerful antioxidant properties and helps to lower cholesterol levels in two ways: It improves the ability of the liver to break down and eliminate cholesterol and it blocks the reabsorption of cholesterol from the intestinal tract into the bloodstream. Turmeric also helps to prevent blood-platelet clumping that can cause dangerous blood clots. Add turmeric liberally to your cooking (it adds a warm, aromatic flavor to soups, curries, salad dressings, and tofu dishes). If you have atherosclerosis, you might want to take larger amounts of turmeric, up to three teaspoons per day, mixed into a small amount of water or juice. Note that turmeric stains deep yellow anything it comes into contact with.

Gugulipid *(Commiphora mukul)* is used in Ayurvedic medicine for treating atherosclerosis and is comparable in effectiveness to cholesterol-lowering drugs but without the negative side effects. It increases the liver's ability to metabolize LDL cholesterol, lowers triglyceride levels, and increases beneficial HDL levels. Gugulipid may also help to rid the arteries of cholesterol buildup. Take gugulipid as a standardized extract, one 500 milligram tablet that contains 25 milligrams of guggulsterone three times a day.

Lifestyle Suggestions for Preventing Atherosclerosis

Regular aerobic exercise is essential for preventing and relieving atherosclerosis. Aerobic activity has clearly been proven to decrease levels of harmful LDL cholesterol and triglycerides and to increase beneficial HDL cholesterol. In addition, exercise strengthens the heart muscle and improves blood supply to the heart. Any type of exercise that moderately increases your heart rate and breathing for a sustained period of time—such as brisk walking, swimming, skiing, dancing, or tennis—will improve your cardiovascular health. Plan for at least 30 minutes of exercise 5 days a week. Try to get outside as much as possible when exercising—sunlight (in reasonable amounts) helps your body to metabolize cholesterol and lowers cholesterol levels. Regular exercise also helps to defuse emotional stress, which plays a significant role in cardiovascular disease.

The well-documented type-A personality, characterized by a chronic sense of time urgency, impatience, and aggressiveness is linked to an increased risk of heart disease. Although we tend to think primarily of men as being driven by type-A personality traits, the truth is that many women also fall into this personality profile. If you suffer from "hurry sickness," do whatever you need to do to learn to let go. Consciously slow down in life, and cultivate patience and a sense of humor. Anxiety and emotional stress also increase your risk of heart disease. Learn to accept those things in life over which you do not have control, and focus your energy where you can make a difference, which most of the time will be right in your own backyard. Cultivate peace of mind. That may sound simplistic, but you really can make a difference in your physiological and psychological health by deciding to be peaceful instead of agitated. For a more thorough treatment of anxiety and stress, see Chapter 13. Many times, physiological problems with the heart have a psychological component of emotional blockage—simply put, the heart is closed on some level. Make time in your life for joy, love, and close relationships, and above all, be compassionate with yourself.

One of the best ways for learning to consciously relax is to set aside time every day to practice relaxation. Choose a method that appeals to you; it might be meditation, yoga, deep relaxation or breathing exercises. See Appendix II for suggestions, and enjoy exploring the options that are available to you. Be sure to also get plenty of sleep and rest, which helps to keep your body functioning optimally and relieves unnecessary stress on your cardiovascular system.

Ellen is a successful magazine editor and loves her work, but 20 years of deadlines have taken a toll on her health. Heart disease runs in her family, but she never gave it much thought—she was too busy building her career, and besides, she felt fine. It was only after a physical exam at age 49 that showed her cholesterol levels had risen to a dangerous high of 240 mg/dl and her blood pressure was 145/90 that she realized she needed to pay serious attention to her health. Ellen began walking for 30 minutes after work, which she found gave her the added benefit of time to unwind after a stressful day. She cut back on saturated fats and eliminated hydrogenated fats and refined supermarket oils from her diet. She started eating salmon and halibut three times a week, garlic every day, and supplemented her diet with a multivitamin and mineral, extra antioxidants, and an herbal extract of hawthorne. In addition, she took high doses of niacin for three months. Ellen's cholesterol and blood pressure began dropping within weeks, and after three months were well within healthy, normal limits. These positive results have motivated her to make even more healthful changes in her life, and she has taken up yoga and meditation to help her maintain a relaxed, more balanced approach to life.

Chapter 24

How to Handle Hypertension

Hypertension, more commonly known as high blood pressure, is the most common chronic medical condition. Normal blood pressure is considered to be 120/80, but the reality is that blood pressure varies continually. Your arteries are meant to be flexible, with the ability to accommodate blood-pressure changes in response to your body's needs. For example, when you are calm and at rest, your blood pressure is naturally lower than when you are tense or active. Blood pressure increases above normal levels when too much blood is being pumped through the blood vessels, or when the blood vessels constrict, which restricts blood flow and increases pressure on the heart and blood vessels. Your blood-pressure reading is a measurement of the pressure that your blood exerts on the walls of your arteries. Each time your heart pumps, it forces blood through your arteries to travel throughout your body. The top number of a blood-pressure reading indicates the amount of pressure on your arteries during a heartbeat (systolic pressure) and the bottom number of a blood-pressure reading indicates the pressure on your arteries when your heart is resting between beats (diastolic pressure).

The range of normal blood pressure is actually somewhere between 85/60 to 135/90. A diagnosis of high blood pressure is made when blood pressure readings are consistently more than 140/90 for a month or two. Even if your blood pressure is elevated, you probably won't feel any symptoms. That's why hypertension is often referred to as the "silent killer." Chronic high blood pressure overworks the heart and damages the blood-vessel walls and greatly increases the risk of heart disease, stroke, kidney damage, and glaucoma. Drugs are commonly prescribed for treating hypertension, but studies show that taking blood-pressure-lowering drugs *increases* the risk of heart disease. Not only can they cause unpleasant side effects such as fatigue and dizziness, but they elevate levels of harmful LDL cholesterol and trigylcerides while decreasing levels of protective HDL cholesterol. The diuretic drugs that are often prescribed can dangerously deplete the body of electrolytes, minerals that naturally lower blood pressure and help to prevent heart attacks. The vast majority of the time, there is no physiological cause for hypertension, and making simple changes in your diet and lifestyle to control blood pressure is clearly a better choice than using drugs.

Lifestyle changes such as eating more healthfully, losing excess weight, exercising regularly, and managing stress are all proven methods of reducing hypertension. In addition, there are a number of dietary supplements and herbs that help to lower high blood pressure and at the same time, strengthen the cardiovascular system. If you have been diagnosed with hypertension, be sure to have your health practitioner check your blood pressure regularly, and learn to monitor your blood pressure yourself so that you can keep track of your progress.

Change Your Diet to Lower Your Blood Pressure

What you eat has a significant effect on your blood-pressure levels. Too much caffeine, alcohol, sugar, saturated fats, and sodium, and too little potassium, calcium, magnesium, vitamin C, fiber, and essential fatty acids lay the groundwork for the development of hypertension. Maintaining healthy arteries is essential for maintaining normal blood pressure, because when the arteries accumulate fatty plaque and become rigid, blood pressure increases. Follow the guidelines for preventing atherosclerosis in Chapter 23.

Sodium is often singled out as the dietary cause of hypertension, but it's not the only factor, and for most people, it's probably not the most important one. However, too much salt can increase blood pressure, particularly if you are sodium sensitive. This doesn't mean that you should completely avoid salt, because it is a necessary mineral that plays a key role in regulating fluid balance in your cells. But most of us get far more sodium than we need. Cutting back on salt is easy if you avoid processed foods—most provide an overdose of sodium in the form of salt or related sodium compounds such as monosodium glutamate. In cooking, you can generally cut the salt called for in recipes in half, and you won't notice the difference. Learn to use liberal amounts of herbs and spices in cooking; not only do they add depth of flavor, but they also contribute valuable trace nutrients and protective antioxidant compounds.

A deficiency of potassium is just as critical as an excess of sodium as a cause of high blood pressure. Low levels of potassium cause the cells to retain too much sodium, which increases fluid retention and raises blood pressure. Potassium also helps to keep all of the muscles, including the heart, contracting and relaxing properly. Avoid processed and canned foods, which tend to be high in sodium and low in potassium, and eat more fresh vegetables and fruits. Foods that are especially rich in potassium include apples, avocados, bananas, oranges, tomatoes, peas, and potatoes.

Other dietary factors that contribute to hypertension include caffeine and alcohol, which cause blood pressure to rise by triggering the release of the stress hormone adrenaline. Avoid alcohol and all sources of caffeine, including chocolate, black tea, coffee-flavored foods, and over-the-counter drugs that contain caffeine or other stimulants. Sugar and refined carbohydrates also act as stimulants, because they trigger the release of adrenaline and insulin. These hormones signal the cells to retain sodium, which increases fluid retention and raises blood pressure. Choose complex carbohydrates in place of refined carbohydrates and fresh fruits instead of refined sugars.

Your easiest solution for lowering high blood pressure is found in your garden or in the produce section of your supermarket.

Recent research shows that eating nine to ten servings of fresh fruits and vegetables a day lowers blood pressure *as effectively* as prescription drugs. That might sound like a lot to crowd into one day's meal planning, but when you consider that one piece of fruit, one-half cup of vegetables, or one cup of leafy greens constitutes a serving, it's not really too difficult. For example, you could eat an orange and one-half of a banana with breakfast, an apple for a midmorning snack, a large bowl of fresh vegetable soup or a large salad with mixed vegetables for lunch, raw carrots for an afternoon snack, and a baked potato and a generous portion of steamed broccoli with dinner. Fresh fruits and vegetables are rich sources of blood-pressure lowering nutrients such as potassium, calcium, magnesium, fiber, and vitamin C and add to your overall well-being in innumerable ways.

If you have hypertension, it's worth cultivating an appreciation for celery. Celery has long been used in Chinese medicine as a treatment for high blood pressure because it relaxes the smooth muscles of the artery walls. For optimum results, you need to eat about four stalks of celery per day. Other vegetables that play an important role in reducing blood pressure are members of the allium family, especially garlic and onions. They contain sulfur compounds, which give them their pungent odor and also their medicinal value. When eaten regularly, they help to relax the blood vessels and also decrease levels of blood fats. Use garlic and onions liberally in your daily cooking, and try also to eat some raw. To help to lower blood pressure and for general cardiovascular health, eat at least one clove of garlic every day, or one-half of an onion.

The omega-3 fatty acids found in cold-water fish and flaxseeds help not only to prevent atherosclerosis, but also to lower high blood pressure. Eat cold-water fish such as salmon, sardines, halibut, tuna, or mackerel two to three times a week, and take one tablespoon of flaxseed oil daily. Flaxseed oil is excellent as a salad dressing or used in place of butter on baked potatoes or pasta.

Supplements That Reduce Blood Pressure

In addition to dietary changes, the following supplements are helpful for bringing blood pressure into a healthful range.

- Vitamin C significantly helps to lower blood pressure, which may partially explain why eating an abundance of fruits and vegetables is so effective for relieving hypertension. In addition to including fruits and vegetables high in vitamin C in your diet (such as citrus fruits, strawberries, red bell peppers, and broccoli), take 2,000 milligrams of vitamin C daily, divided into two or three doses.

- Magnesium, along with potassium and sodium, is essential for regulating fluid balance in the cells. Most people get too much sodium in their diets and not enough potassium and magnesium. Because potassium is abundant in fresh fruits and vegetables, as well as nuts, soybeans, and fish, supplements are rarely required. Magnesium is found in whole grains, raw nuts and seeds, and legumes, but most women fall far short of the daily requirement for optimal health. Include plenty of magnesium-rich foods in your diet, and take 400 to 600 milligrams of magnesium citrate, aspartate, gluconate, or lactate daily.

- Calcium helps to prevent the development of high blood pressure and also helps to lower high blood pressure caused by sodium sensitivity. Eat calcium-rich foods such as yogurt, tofu, sardines, sesame seeds, almonds, and dark-leafy greens, and take 1,000 milligrams daily of calcium citrate, aspartate, lactate, gluconate, or malate, with meals.

- Coenzyme Q-10 helps to alleviate hypertension and also helps to protect the heart and the arteries from damage caused by high blood pressure. To help to prevent high blood pressure and protect the cardiovascular system, take 30 to 60 milligrams per day of CoQ-10 in gel capsules. If you have hypertension, take 120 milligrams twice daily.

Relieve Hypertension with Herbs

The powerful cardiovascular tonic herbs garlic and hawthorne (discussed on page 224) form the basis of an herbal-treatment program for preventing and alleviating hypertension.

Hawthorne helps to lower blood pressure by dilating the arteries, which improves blood flow and prevents the arterial tension that raises blood-pressure levels. As little as one clove of *garlic* per day lowers both cholesterol and blood-pressure levels. Mild diuretic herbs such as *dandelion, linden,* and *yarrow,* are helpful because they reduce total blood volume, which also lowers blood pressure. If anxiety and stress are a contributing factor, see Chapter 13 for appropriate herbal recommendations.

Dandelion *(Taraxacum officinale)* leaves are as effective as the pharmaceutical diuretics prescribed for hypertension but without the harmful side effects. Because dandelion leaves are rich in potassium, there is not the danger of creating electrolyte imbalances that can cause heart-rate disturbances. Dandelion has a bitter, but not unpleasant taste. To make a tea from dandelion, pour one cup of boiling water over two teaspoons of dried leaf, cover, and steep for 15 minutes.

Linden *(Tilia x vulgaris)* is also a mild diuretic and is excellent in combination with other herbs for treating high blood pressure. Because it helps to calm the nervous system, it is especially helpful for relieving hypertension that is related to emotional stress. Linden flower tea has a delicate, pleasant flavor. Pour one cup of boiling water over two teaspoons of dried herb, cover, and steep for 15 minutes. Strain and drink up to three cups daily.

Yarrow *(Achillea millefolium)* helps to lower blood pressure by dilating the peripheral blood vessels and also through its mild diuretic properties. It has a bitter, aromatic flavor. To make a tea, pour one cup of boiling water over two teaspoons of dried yarrow, cover, and steep for 15 minutes. Strain, and drink up to three cups a day.

Herbal Tea for Hypertension

3 teaspoons hawthorne berries or flowers
3 teaspoons linden
2 teaspoons yarrow
3 cups water

Pour three cups of boiling water over dried herbs, cover, and steep for 20 minutes. Strain, and drink 3 cups a day. You can also make this formula as a liquid extract by combining prepared extracts in the same proportions. Take 1 teaspoon 3 times a day with a small amount of warm water.

Lifestyle Changes for Lowering Blood Pressure

Exercise is a key component of a natural approach to lowering blood pressure. Regular moderate aerobic exercise helps to directly alleviate hypertension and also reduces the emotional stress that contributes to elevated blood-pressure levels. Spend at least 30 minutes five times a week in activities that gently increase your heart rate and breathing, such as brisk walking, hiking, bicycling, or dancing.

Meditative forms of exercise such as yoga and tai chi are also excellent for relieving high blood pressure. They help to regulate breathing and heart rate, and reduce levels of stress hormones that contribute to hypertension. Deep-relaxation exercises and meditation will do the same, and if practiced even for a few minutes daily can be remarkably effective at lowering blood-pressure levels. See Appendix II for suggestions for relaxation exercises.

Reducing the emotional stress in your life is critical for relieving high blood pressure. Eliminate stress triggers if possible; but even more important is to change the way that you respond to life stressors. Learn to slow down, to relax, and to take life with more gentleness and humor. High blood pressure can also be related to emotions that you keep bottled up inside. Try journaling or talking with a trusted friend to keep internal pressure from building. Psychotherapy can be immensely helpful for providing a safe space for unraveling deeply held tension. See Chapter 13 for more information on stress and anxiety.

Aromatherapy Help for Hypertension

While aromatherapy is not a cure for hypertension, essential oils can help to ease the physical and emotional tension that contribute to elevated blood-pressure levels. Try using essential oils regularly in a bath or a massage. Add approximately 15 drops of lavender or marjoram to a tub of warm water and two drops of ylang ylang if desired. Soak for 15–20 minutes, allowing yourself to deeply relax.

Lavender is balancing and soothing for both the body and the mind and has relaxing and blood-pressure-lowering effects. It has a sweet, herbaceous floral fragrance.

Marjoram is an excellent sedative. It helps to ease muscle tension, dilates the peripheral arteries, and lowers blood pressure. It has a warm, herbaceous, slightly sweet fragrance with undertones of camphor.

Ylang-ylang has potent sedative properties and helps to regulate cardiovascular function and lower blood pressure. It has an intensely sweet, floral scent. Use in moderation—a drop or two at most is sufficient. In excess, ylang-ylang can cause headaches.

Massage Oil for Hypertension

4 ounces almond oil

20 drops lavender essential oil

15 drops marjoram essential oil

2 drops ylang-ylang essential oil

1 teaspoon vitamin E oil

Combine almond oil, essential oils and vitamin E oil in a dark-glass bottle. Store in a cool, dark place, and shake well before using.

Chapter 25

Strengthen Your Immune System to Prevent Cancer

Although modern medicine has been promising for decades to win the war on cancer, the battle is far from over. It may be an impossible task, because cancer appears in so many different forms, and it is unlikely that any one "magic-bullet" treatment will ever eradicate the disease. The good news is that your body is programmed to prevent cancer from developing, and there are many steps you can take to strengthen your body's natural resistance.

Cancer doesn't happen overnight; it can take 20 years or more to develop. We generate cancerous cells throughout our lives, and it is the job of the immune system to search out and destroy cells that have gone astray. Specialized white blood cells constantly patrol the body, looking for cancerous cells. When they find an abnormal cell, they engulf and kill it before it can reproduce. The body has another built-in protection against cancer: Any cell that begins to multiply out of control is programmed to commit suicide, a process called apoptosis. Most of the time, the body's protective systems work well. But if you are exposed to large amounts of cancer-causing substances, cancer cells can multiply more rapidly than the immune system can destroy them, or the immune system may become defective in its ability to recognize and destroy cancerous cells.

Cancer appears in many different forms, but all types of cancer have some characteristics in common. They reproduce more rapidly than the cells from which they originated, and they bear little resemblance to those original cells. Unlike normal cells, they also invade neighboring tissues and spread to other areas of the body where they begin to multiply and grow into tumors. The development of cancer is generally a long, slow process that is triggered by cellular damage caused by free radicals. (A free radical is a molecule missing an electron that steals an electron from a healthy molecule, creating a new free radical and setting up a chain reaction of cellular damage.) To prevent cancer, you can protect your cells from free-radical damage in two ways: You can reduce your exposure to toxins, and you can strengthen the resistance of your cells.

Our immune systems are our first line of defense against the development of cancerous cells. But our immune systems are under great stress today because of the thousands of toxic chemicals we encounter in our environment, food, and water. To magnify the problem, the typical diet is deficient in the essential nutrients that keep the immune system healthy.

How to Avoid Weakening Your Immune System

Environmental toxins, radiation, viruses, and physical irritants can all cause cancer by permanently altering the DNA of a cell. The DNA is like a cellular blueprint that tells each individual cell how to perfectly reproduce itself. Malignant changes are bound to happen, because there are ten million cells replaced every second in our bodies. Every mutation does not cause cancer, however, because the immune system is constantly on the lookout for malignant cells and immediately eliminates them. For cancer to arise, the immune system has to fail at its job. The best way to prevent cancer is to do all that you can to keep your immune system functioning optimally.

There are specific protective steps you can take to keep from harming your immune system. Avoid exposure to radiation as much as possible, including diagnostic X-rays unless they are absolutely necessary. Radiation causes damage to DNA that is cumulative over a lifetime. Because every exposure to toxins also increases the possibility of malignant changes in your cells, no encounter with toxins is without harm. Your liver is responsible for detoxifying and neutralizing all of the chemicals that you come into contact with as well as toxins that are generated by normal metabolic processes. The vast amount of toxins that most of us encounter every day places a tremendous burden on the liver. When your liver is overburdened, toxins accumulate in your body and compromise the health of your immune system. To protect your liver, avoid poisonous chemicals such as pesticides, herbicides, tobacco, over-the-counter and prescription drugs, food additives, and household and garden chemicals. In addition, you can take herbs such as *milk thistle, tumeric,* and *licorice root* to protect and rejuvenate your liver.

Milk thistle *(Silybum marianum)* is a powerful herb that protects the liver from being damaged by toxins and actually helps to regenerate the liver. The active ingredient, silymarin, is a potent antioxidant that prevents free-radical damage to the liver. In addition, silymarin stimulates the production of healthy new liver cells and helps the liver to detoxify toxic chemicals by increasing levels of the body's own protective antioxidant, glutathione. Take a standardized extract of milk thistle that provides 140 milligrams of silymarin three times a day. A standardized extract ensures that you are getting adequate amounts of the active ingredients, but you can also use milk thistle seed in a tea or add a tablespoon or two of ground milk thistle seeds to cereal or salads. The seeds have a hard coating and must be ground to access their healing properties. To make a tea, steep two teaspoons of the ground seeds in one cup of boiling water for 15 minutes. Strain, and drink three cups a day.

Turmeric *(Curcuma longa)* has been valued in Ayurvedic medicine for centuries as a whole-body cleansing herb. It has powerful antioxidant properties and protects cells against the formation of carcinogens, as well as enhancing levels of glutathione, one of the most potent natural antioxidants produced by the body. Turmeric has been shown to inhibit cancer and may even help to promote the regression of existing cancers. The antioxidant action of turmeric protects the liver against toxins, and the bitter components stimulate liver cleansing by enhancing bile production. Turmeric is best absorbed when taken with meals containing some fat. The warm, fragrant flavor of turmeric is excellent in soups, curries, and grain dishes. You can also stir one-half to one teaspoon of turmeric into water or juice and take it two to three times a day with a meal.

Licorice *(Glycyrrhiza glabra)* improves liver function by preventing free-radical damage as well as by inhibiting the formation of free radicals. It contains natural compounds called glycyrrhizin and glycyrrhetinic acid, which are easily absorbed into the bloodstream, where they enhance immune function. In large doses, however, these same compounds can cause fluid retention in susceptible people. You can prevent the possible side effects of licorice by increasing your potassium intake and decreasing your sodium intake. However, do not use licorice daily for more than one month without checking with your health practioner, and if you have high blood pressure or cardiovascular or kidney disease, consult your health practitioner before using licorice root. To prepare licorice tea, simmer one-half to one teaspoon of licorice root in one cup of water in a covered pot for 10 minutes. Strain, and drink up to three cups a day. Licorice has an extremely sweet flavor, which makes it a welcome addition to herbal-tea blends.

Guidelines for Strengthening Immune Function

Your immune system is the most complex system of your body, and scientists are still uncovering new insights about how the organs, glands, and cells function together to keep you in optimal health. The primary job of your immune system is to protect your body against infectious microorganisms and to prevent the development of cancer. Your immune system is constantly on patrol, checking cells for evidence of infection and looking for cells that show cancerous changes.

Your immune system has many different components and is spread throughout your body. Your thymus gland (found at the base of your neck), spleen (located just under your rib cage on the left side of your body), bone marrow, and a large network of lymph nodes (including your tonsils) make up the basic structure of your immune system. Hundreds of lymph nodes are scattered throughout your body and are concentrated primarily in your armpits, neck, groin, abdomen, and chest. Your immune system also contains a variety of white blood cells including natural-killer cells (white blood cells that destroy cancerous cells) that circulate throughout the blood and lymphatic fluid, looking for infectious microorganisms and diseased cells. In addition, your immune system contains specialized immune cells called macrophages that gobble up diseased or damaged cells, and other special compounds such as interferon, interleukin II, and complement fractions that stimulate white blood cells to destroy cancer cells.

Strengthening your immune system is critical for preventing the development of cancer, because it is your first line of defense against the cellular changes that lead to cancer. If your immune system is not functioning up to par, not only are you more likely to come down with frequent infections, but you are also at higher risk for cancer. If you catch colds easily or come down with more than one or two colds per year or if you have any type of chronic infection (such as a recurring yeast infection), your immune system is not functioning as well as it could be. Here are the primary ways that you can enhance your immunity, which will strengthen your resistance to cancer:

- **Eat a nutrient-rich diet.** Nutrient deficiencies are a primary cause of depressed immunity. Eat a diet centered around fresh vegetables and fruits, grains, legumes, nuts, and seeds—they are concentrated sources of nutrients and provide cell-protecting antioxidants. Adequate amounts of high-quality proteins are essential for optimal immune function; eat six to eight ounces of fish, chicken, tofu, or other balanced protein foods daily. Avoid food grown or prepared with chemicals and commercially produced meats and dairy foods, because they often contain residues of antibiotics that are harmful to the immune system. Don't eat polyunsaturated, hydrogenated, or partially hydrogenated oils because they create free radicals that can hinder immune function. Avoid sugar and all concentrated sweeteners (including excessive amounts of fruit juice) because even one sugary treat significantly lowers your immune defenses for several hours.

- **Exercise regularly.** Exercising four to five times a week for 30 minutes at a time has been proven to boost immune function. You can exercise more if you like, but avoid overly strenuous exercise (such as marathon running) because it lowers your immune function. The number of all types of white blood cells increases with moderate exercise, and natural killer cells become more effective. It's even better if you find some form of exercise that you truly love, because your immune function is further enhanced when you enjoy what you do.

- **Reduce stress in your life.** Emotional stress and unresolved emotions inhibit immunity. Your emotional state has a measurable effect on your immune system. Emotional stress stimulates the secretion of adrenal hormones such as adrenaline and corticosteroids, which have a suppressive effect on the white blood cells and thymus gland. When you are depressed, your immunity also plummets. Even a simple process of journaling about upsetting incidents has been proven to improve immune function. Take 20 minutes every day to write about whatever is on your mind, including any events that have upset you at any time in your life that still tug at you emotionally. Include as many details as you can about the incident, as well as all your feelings. Giving yourself the opportunity to get your feelings down on paper helps to free you from carrying around unresolved pain, anger, and grief. You may also want to work with a therapist if you feel that emotional pain is holding you back and getting in the way of your living fully and enjoying life. For more suggestions for relieving stress and depression, see Chapters 13 and 14.

- **Make relationships a priority.** The quality of your relationships has a powerful influence on your immune function. People who have close, meaningful relationships are happier than those who are isolated, and they have stronger immune systems. Make sure that you make time in your life every day for relationships that you enjoy.

- **Get enough sleep.** Try to get at least seven hours per night or more of sleep, because your immune system is dependent on sufficient sleep to work properly. A lack of sleep impairs immune function, affecting the production of lymphocytes, natural-killer cells, and macrophage activity. In addition, powerful immune-enhancing compounds are released during deep, restful sleep. If you have problems sleeping, see Chapter 15 for suggestions.

- **Don't allow infections to linger.** Treat any infection such as a respiratory infection promptly with immune-boosting herbs such as *echinacea* and *astragalus,* get plenty of rest, and do all you can to help your body overcome the infection. Infections tax the immune system, and chronic or recurrent infections such as gum or tooth infections can significantly inhibit immunity. Whenever possible, however, avoid using antibiotics to treat infections, because they ultimately weaken immune function. Save antibiotics for infections that cannot be easily or safely treated with natural herbal alternatives such as echinacea, astragalus, garlic, and goldenseal.

- **Avoid exposure to toxins.** Limit your exposure to radiation, and to all types of toxic chemicals because they impair immune function and contribute to the formation of cell-damaging free radicals.

Enhance Your Immunity with Herbal Tonics

Western medicine is just now beginning to recognize the wisdom of enhancing the body's innate ability for self-protection and healing. Traditional Chinese medicine has always focused on strengthening the *wei chi,* the protective energy of the body, and over the centuries has developed an herbal repertoire of powerful immune-enhancing herbs. Some of the most revered remedies in Chinese medicine are mushrooms that are used as tonics to strengthen the body, increase resistance to disease, and promote longevity.

Although we tend to think of mushrooms primarily as ingredients for creating gourmet meals, traditional doctors in the Orient hold medicinal mushrooms in high regard for their healing properties. The primary active compounds in medicinal mushrooms appear to be polysaccharides—large, complex sugar molecules that stimulate immune function and have anticancer properties. Many of these valuable mushrooms grow wild and are difficult to find; their use in ancient times was reserved only for those who had the money or status to obtain them. Fortunately, these same mushrooms are now successfully being cultivated in this country and are some of the most powerful immune tonics available. Take any or all of these tonics as desired to strengthen your immune function. They all are safe to use over an extended period of time and can be thought of as nourishment for your immune system.

Shiitake *(Lentinula edodes)* is a Japanese mushroom with a rich, meaty flavor that has been valued for centuries for its ability to enhance vitality. Shiitake contains at least one anticancer substance called lentinan, which has been proven to improve immune function, including increasing the production of interferon and other important immune compounds. You can find fresh shiitake in many supermarkets, and they are also widely available dried. Shiitake are a flavorful addition to soups, stir-fries, and pasta dishes. For immune enhancement, eat a few shiitake at least a couple of times a week.

Maitake *(Grifola frondosa)* is a delicious mushroom that grows in clusters that look like the ruffled tail feathers of a hen, hence the common name "hen of the woods." Maitake increases cellular immunity and inhibits cancerous growths, and scientists have proven that an extract from this mushroom directly activates various cells of the immune system, including macrophages and natural-killer cells. Maitake is sold dried for use in cooking and teas and is available fresh in some markets. It's also sold as a concentrated extract, either as a whole extract or as maitake d-fraction extract. Eat fresh or dried reconstituted maitake a couple of times a week in soups, stir-fries, and pasta dishes, or take approximately 10 to 20 drops of the extract twice daily.

Astragalus *(Astragalus membranaceous)* is not a mushroom, but a member of the legume family, and the fibrous root is one of the most powerful immune-enhancing herbs known. Astragalus stimulates the body's natural-defense mechanisms, including enhancing the activity of macrophages and natural-killer cells. It has been proven effective in increasing resistance to a wide spectrum of immune-system breakdowns, from the common cold to cancer, and is also helpful for restoring immune function that has been damaged as a result of chemotherapy or radiation treatment. Astragalus has a pleasant, slightly sweet, earthy flavor. It is available either dried and shredded, or in the traditional form of dried slices (they look like tongue depressors) that you find in Chinese herb stores. The shredded form is easier to use for making tea, and the dried slices are easier to use in soup because astragalus is very fibrous and, after simmering, must be removed from the soup.

Immune Tonic Tea

3 tablespoons shredded astragalus root
2 teaspoons licorice root
2 teaspoons chopped fresh ginger root

Simmer astragalus, licorice, and ginger in 3 1/2 cups of water for 20 minutes. Strain, and drink up to 3 cups daily.

Immune-Building Tonic Soup

1 ounce sliced dried astragalus root
1 inch fresh ginger root, slivered
1/2 cup brown basmati rice
1/4 teaspoon sea salt
6–8 cups vegetable or chicken stock
2 tablespoons extra-virgin olive oil
1/2 cup onions, chopped
1/2 cup carrots, sliced into half-moons
1/2 cup fresh shiitake mushrooms, sliced (or 1/4 cup dried)
1/2 cup fresh maitake mushrooms, sliced (or 1/4 cup dried)
6 cloves garlic, minced
1/4 cup light miso
1/4 cup parsley, minced

1. *Simmer the astragalus, ginger, rice, sea salt, and stock in a heavy, covered pot for 1 hour. If you are using dried shiitake and maitake, include them at the same time.*

2. *Sauté the onions, carrots, shiitake, and maitake (if you are using fresh mushrooms) in olive oil for 5 minutes. Add the garlic, and saute for 1 minute.*

3. *Add the sautéed vegetable mixture to the soup pot, cover, and simmer for 30 minutes. Remove the astragalus slices.*

4. *Dilute the miso with a small amount of hot broth and add to the soup along with the parsley. Remove from heat, cover, and let stand for 5 minutes before serving.*

Six Dietary Steps to Prevent Cancer

The foods you eat on a daily basis are clearly linked to your risk of cancer—at least one-third of all cancers are directly caused by dietary factors. While many foods are known to contribute to cancer, there are just as many foods that prevent cancer. Use the following six steps to create a diet that is rich in protective nutrients.

   1. Eat a wide variety of fresh fruits and vegetables, at least five servings per day, and preferably nine or more. Fresh fruits and vegetables are rich in fiber, vitamins, and minerals, as well as in a variety of antioxidants and other protective compounds called phytochemicals that help to protect cells from damage and block the growth of cancerous cells. A serving is one-half cup of fruit, one-half cup of cooked vegetable, one cup of leafy greens, one average size piece of fruit, one-quarter cup of dried fruit, or six ounces of fresh fruit or vegetable juice. Vary the fruits and vegetables you eat every day to get a wide range of protective nutrients, and buy organic produce to avoid harmful pesticides and herbicides. A simple way to ensure that you are getting a variety of protective nutrients is to include an array of different colors of fruits and vegetables in your diet—try to eat something red, yellow, orange, green, and purple every day.

- Cruciferous vegetables such as broccoli, cabbage, cauliflower, bok choy, kale, mustard greens, watercress, and brussels sprouts contain a variety of cancer-fighting substances, including sulfur compounds called indoles, that help to convert estrogen from a potentially carcinogenic form to a form that has cancer-protective properties. Other substances in cruciferous vegetables increase the production of the body's natural antioxidant compound glutathione, which helps to neutralize carcinogens.

- Members of the allium family such as garlic, onions, scallions, leeks, shallots, and chives are rich in the antioxidant selenium and enhance the activity of immune cells that fight cancer, as well as increasing levels of enzymes that break down carcinogens. It probably comes as no surprise that garlic is the most powerful member of the allium family; to help protect your cells against cancer, eat one clove of garlic every day.

- Vitamin-C-rich fruits and vegetables such as citrus fruits, strawberries, kiwi, broccoli, and red peppers prevent free radicals from damaging cells and causing the mutations that lead to cancer.

- Fruits and vegetables high in beta-carotene neutralize free radicals, improve immune function, and even help to reverse precancerous changes in cells. Beta-carotene is abundant in deep yellow and orange fruits and vegetables such as carrots, sweet potatoes, yams, winter squashes, cantaloupe, and apricots, and in dark-green vegetables such as broccoli, collards, and kale.

- Lycopene is a potent cancer preventative phytochemical found in tomatoes, watermelon, red peppers, and carrots.

- Oranges, lemons, and limes contain a phytochemical called limonene that raises levels of enzymes that help to break down carcinogens and also stimulates immune cells that eradicate cancer.

- Grapes, apples, strawberries, and raspberries contain ellagic acid, a phytochemical that blocks the body's production of enzymes used by cancer cells and helps to slow tumor growth.

- Glutathione is a potent antioxidant that plays a critical role in detoxification. Glutathione helps to neutralize and break down free radicals so that they can be eliminated by the body. Asparagus, broccoli, cauliflower, grapefruit, onions, oranges, potatoes, tomatoes, and watermelon are rich in glutathione.

    2. Limit your fat intake to no more than 20 to 30 percent of your daily calories. Diets high in saturated fats, polyunsaturated oils, and hydrogenated oils greatly increase cancer risk by generating large numbers of dangerous free radicals. A high-fat diet also creates chemicals in the intestinal tract that are converted by bacteria to harmful estrogens that trigger reproductive and breast cancers. The kinds of fats you eat may be even more important than the amount. Avoid saturated fats, found in red meat, full-fat dairy products, and palm and coconut oils. Polyunsaturated oils such as safflower, corn, soybean, and sunflower oils are extremely detrimental to your health because they are unstable and oxidize rapidly, creating free radicals. The most harmful of the toxic fats are hydrogenated or partially hydrogenated oils, which mutate into a particularly dangerous compound known as transfatty acids during processing. They are loaded with free radicals and once inside your body continue to oxidize and generate more free radicals.

Although fat in general has gotten bad press, some fats, such as extra-virgin olive oil, actually protect your cells against cancer. Olive oil is a monounsaturated oil and slow to oxidize. In addition, it makes cell membranes more resistant to the destructive effects of free radicals thereby helping to prevent cancer. Cultures that eat large amounts of olive oil, such as Spain, have much lower cancer rates than do other Western countries.

3. **Eat plenty of fiber in the form of whole grains, legumes, nuts, seeds, vegetables, and fruits.** Fiber helps to move wastes more quickly through the intestinal tract, shortening the time that toxins remain in the body. Fiber also helps to reduce circulating levels of estrogen by binding to estrogen in the intestinal tract and preventing it from reentering the bloodstream. Try to eat about 35 grams of fiber every day. Cooked dried legumes such as kidney beans are excellent sources of fiber with more than seven grams per half-cup serving. Most fruits and vegetables contain about three grams of fiber per average serving. If you need extra fiber, boost your intake with fiber supplements such as psyllium and pectin.

4. **Include omega-3 rich fatty acids in your diet, found in cold-water fish and flaxseeds.** Omega-3 fatty acids inhibit hormone-like compounds called prostaglandins which cause inflammation and interfere with the immune system's ability to detect and destroy cancerous cells. Omega-3 fatty acids also help to block the development and spread of cancer. While a high consumption of animal fats is linked to a higher incidence of cancer, a high consumption of fish is associated with a lower incidence of cancer. It's interesting to note that North American Eskimo women, who eat a diet incredibly rich in omega-3 fatty acids, have *no* breast cancer whatsoever.

Cold-water fish that are good sources of omega-3 fatty acids include salmon, mackerel, sardines, halibut, and fresh tuna. To protect your cells against cancer, eat two to three servings of cold-water fish weekly. Flaxseeds are a good vegetarian source of omega-3 fatty acids, and they also contain compounds called lignans, which bind to estrogen receptors and help to inhibit the growth of estrogen-dependent cancers. Take one tablespoon of flaxseed oil daily or add one to two tablespoons of freshly ground flaxseeds to cereals or salads. Do not heat flax oil, but use it to make salad dressings, or add it to baked potatoes, vegetables, or pasta.

5. **Eat soy foods such as soybeans, tofu, tempeh, and miso.** Soybeans contain genistein, a natural plant estrogen that binds to the estrogen receptors of hormone-sensitive tissues (such as the breasts) and prevents the more powerful and potentially carcinogenic estrogen made by your body from occupying the sites. Soybeans also contain compounds called protease inhibitors, which block the action of proteases, enzymes that stimulate tumor growth. The potent anticancer compounds found in soyfoods inhibit the development of small blood vessels that provide tumors with oxygen and nutrients, they increase the demise of cancer cells, and they help to break down potential cancer-causing substances in the body. Eat four ounces of soy foods daily, preferably those that are made in the more traditional forms (tofu, tempeh, miso, and whole soybeans) instead of soy luncheon meats, cheeses, and other highly processed products.

6. **Drink green tea, at least three cups per day.** Green tea contains potent antioxidants called polyphenols which inhibit free-radical damage to cells. It also contains catechins, a type of polyphenol that prevents cancer cells from multiplying and helps the body to eliminate carcinogens. The Japanese habit of drinking numerous cups of green tea every day is thought to be associated with their significantly lower incidence of cancer. Green tea is an excellent substitute for coffee or black tea and provides a mild energizing boost.

Protect Your Cells with Antioxidants

Supplements are not a substitute for a healthful diet, but they can provide insurance protection for your cells. To prevent cancer, it is essential to keep your cells saturated with antioxidants, and it's difficult to obtain sufficient amounts of antioxidants solely through foods. Take a high-potency vitamin-and-mineral supplement daily to provide a wide range of nutrients that act in various ways to prevent cancer. Make sure that you are getting the following range of protective antioxidants, and take extra supplements if necessary to fill the gap:

> **Beta-carotene**—25,000 units daily
>
> **Vitamin C**—2,000 milligrams daily
>
> **Vitamin E**—400–800 units daily
>
> **Selenium**—200 micrograms daily
>
> **Zinc**—30 milligrams daily
>
> **CoQ-10**—30–60 milligrams daily

Living Healthfully to Prevent Cancer

There are many small steps you can take to create a healthful lifestyle that will not only prevent cancer, but will also enhance and enrich your life in many ways. Incorporate as many of these suggestions as you can into your life.

- Get four hours or more of moderately vigorous aerobic exercise every week. Physical activity improves your immune function and increases the circulation of blood and lymph, which helps your body to detoxify. Exercise also relieves stress and elevates your mood, which plays a powerful role in your health. Studies show that women who exercise four hours or more per week have a 60 percent lower risk of breast cancer than do inactive women.

- Although an excessive amount of sun exposure is a primary cause of skin cancer, a moderate amount can help to prevent cancer. Sunshine is necessary for the production of vitamin D, which is linked to lower rates of cancer. Moderate means about 15 minutes of sun daily in the early morning or late afternoon when the sun's rays are not too strong.

- Get plenty of sleep, and make sure that you sleep in total darkness, because light decreases your body's production of the hormone melatonin. Low levels of melatonin are associated with an increased risk of cancer.

- Don't smoke, and don't be exposed to secondhand smoke.

- Avoid excessive amounts of alcohol, more than a few drinks per week. If you are going to drink, choose organic red wine, which has some health benefits. But be aware than any alcohol intake appears to be associated with an increased risk of breast cancer.

- Avoid exposure to all types of environmental toxins, both at home and at work. Buy organic foods, use filtered water, cut back on animal fats and full-fat dairy products because they concentrate toxins and hormones, and avoid using toxic chemicals in your home and garden. Be especially wary of compounds that are called environmental estrogens or endocrine disrupters. They alter hormone function and are associated with an increased risk of cancer, especially reproductive cancers. These compounds are insidious and occur in food and water as residues from pesticides and other chemicals, in conventionally raised meats and dairy products, and in items that you would probably never guess would be highly carcinogenic such as plastic food wrap and plastic containers. The plastic found in many of these items can be absorbed into foods and beverages; that's why water in soft plastic bottles often tastes like plastic. Do not use plastics for cooking or for microwaving and avoid using plastic wrap.

- There appears to be a "cancer-prone personality," described as someone who has difficulty expressing so-called negative feelings such as anger and sadness and who suppresses emotions in order always to be pleasant and agreeable. Suppressed emotions suppress immune function, because your mind, nervous system, and immune system are intricately interwoven. It takes a tremendous amount of psychic and physical energy to keep emotions and traumatic events hidden away. Inner-process work such as journaling, therapy, and body work is immensely helpful for accessing your feelings and your innermost self.

- Meditate or engage in some other form of daily practice that nourishes your spirit. Simply allowing for a few minutes of silent reflection every day helps to bring your body, mind, and spirit into balance.

- Make sure that your life is rich with connections to people who bring love to your life and with whom you can share your deepest thoughts and feelings.

- Add pleasure to your life as much as possible. Look for opportunities to enhance your experience of daily life in small ways, such as having tea with a friend, walking in a beautiful place in nature, reading a good book, planting a garden, or enjoying a delicious meal.

- Practice relaxation exercises every day to help bring your body into balance and to strengthen your immune function. Accumulated stressors create free radicals, and deep-breathing exercises are one of the most powerful tools you have for immediately shifting out of the stress response and into a state of relaxation. See Appendix II for suggestions for relaxation exercises.

How to Eat for Optimal Health

Good nutrition is always essential for good health, but optimal nutrition is essential for optimal health at midlife and beyond. After the age of 40, your body is not likely to be as forgiving of dietary indiscretions and overindulgences as it once was. If you aren't already eating a health-supportive diet, this is the perfect time to begin. What you choose to eat affects not only your daily energy level and mood, but your long-term health as well. Your dietary choices are a critical factor in whether or not you will develop degenerative diseases such as heart disease, cancer, and diabetes, and researchers are discovering almost daily the remarkable benefits of health-enhancing compounds found in natural, unprocessed foods. Eating healthfully does not mean living a life of deprivation. On the contrary—eating is a great sensual pleasure, and cooking and eating well is a wonderful way to nurture yourself. Taking the time and making the effort to eat well isn't always easy, but the rewards are great. Think of it this way—each time you eat, you have the opportunity to improve your health.

A simple way of approaching dietary change is to make your diet nutrient dense. This means evaluating what you eat on the basis of what it offers to you. The foods you eat should be delicious and satisfying and should also supply your body with optimum levels of nutrients that will keep you healthy, strong, and energetic. While it makes sense to educate yourself about foods and nutrients and the role they play in health, it is equally important to pay close attention to how particular foods affect you. We are all unique individuals with different dietary needs. To feel your best, you need to discover the diet that best supports your particular body, genetic makeup, and lifestyle. You may find it helpful to work with a nutritionist or health practitioner who is skilled in nutrition, but ultimately, your best guidance is to listen to your inner wisdom.

About ten years ago, I followed a strict vegan diet for several years because intellectually and philosophically I believed it was the perfect diet. I know people who do just fine on this type of diet, but after about a year of eating no animal products, I was chronically tired, had gained weight, my skin and hair were excessively dry, my joints ached, and I craved sweets intensely—but I didn't associate the limited diet I was eating with my symptoms. During my fourth year of eating a vegan diet, I started having recurring dreams about eating salmon, but I ignored my dreams because eating fish did not fit in with my dietary philosophy. About six months passed, and I started dreaming about eating hamburgers, which I had not eaten for more than 20 years! I suddenly had the realization that my body was desperately trying to communicate with me through my dreams and that perhaps my declining health was related to a diet that wasn't meeting my needs. That night I ate salmon for dinner, and it seemed like exactly the right thing to do. I continued eating fish two to three times a week, my health and energy steadily improved, I effortlessly lost weight, and the vague health concerns that had been bothering me disappeared. It was a tremendous lesson for me in learning to listen to the wisdom of my body.

I encourage you to do the same. Use the following guidelines, not as a restrictive diet, but as a starting point for developing an optimal way of eating that helps you to reach your particular goals of health, vitality, and well-being.

The Four Basic Principles of a Healthful Diet

1. **Eat a diet rich in whole, unrefined, nutrient-dense foods.** Fresh, natural, minimally processed foods are the richest in nutrients, including the trace compounds that are critical for optimal health.

2. **Eat a wide variety of foods.** No one food has a perfect balance of nutrients, and eating a wide variety of foods provides you with a wide variety of nutrients. Most people get into dietary ruts, eating only a handful of foods. Broadening your food choices provides you with a greater abundance of the vitamins, minerals, antioxidants, essential fatty acids, and phytonutrients that support optimal health. In addition, eating a variety of foods decreases the possibility of creating food sensitivities that can arise when the same few foods are eaten day after day.

3. **Avoid foods grown, treated, or processed with chemicals.** Virtually every one of us carry residues of pesticides and other chemicals stored in our body tissues. These poisons enter our food supply in a variety of ways: pesticides and other agricultural chemicals are applied to crops, animals raised for the meat and dairy industries are fed hormones and antibiotics, and a huge array of chemicals are added to foods during processing to flavor, sweeten, color, preserve, and texturize them. Even food packaging contains toxins that leach into the contents, such as lead or aluminum in cans and polyvinyl chloride in plastic food wrap. All chemicals add to the load of poisons that the liver is forced to detoxify and create free-radical damage that leads to cancer, heart disease, other degenerative diseases, and premature aging. Make every effort to buy organically grown and processed foods.

4. **Discover the diet that is best for you.** Take the time to find a way of eating that makes you feel healthy and energetic. Pay attention to how you feel, don't be afraid to experiment, and remember that no one diet is the perfect diet for everyone. For example, although the high-complex carbohydrate, low-fat, and low-protein diet has been popularized as the ultimate healthful way of eating, many women find that a diet consisting primarily of car-

bohydrates—even healthful complex carbohydrates—increases insulin levels and causes fatigue, weight gain, dry skin, and hormonal imbalances. This is particularly true for women over 40. Many women find that eating more protein and fat (healthful fats, of course) makes all the difference in the way they feel. A diet that consists of about 30 percent protein, 30 percent fat, and 40 percent carbohydrates helps to keep blood sugar on an even keel and prostaglandin levels balanced.

Nine Steps to Improving Your Diet

1. **Eat an abundance of fresh vegetables and fruits.** Eating a lot of fresh vegetables and fruits provides a wide range of antioxidants and phytonutrients that help to prevent disease and slow down the aging process. Although the standard current recommendation is to eat five servings daily of fresh fruits and vegetables, an optimal intake is at least seven and preferably nine servings daily. Vegetables and fruits saturate your cells with protective nutrients, and the soluble fiber they contain helps to cleanse the intestinal tract and arteries. For the richest sources of antioxidants and phytonutrients, choose vegetables and fruits with the deepest colors—for example, choose dark-leafy greens over pale lettuces, and purple or red grapes over green grapes.

While raw foods generally have the highest concentrations of beneficial compounds, some nutrients, such as beta-carotene, are more easily absorbed when vegetables are lightly cooked. The best approach is to eat a variety of raw and lightly cooked vegetables. Consider one-half cup of cooked or raw vegetables, one cup of raw leafy greens, one-half cup or one piece of fruit, or one cup of fresh vegetable or fruit juice as one serving. Give vegetables a starring role at lunch and dinner and use them as snacks throughout the day. Fruits provide a natural satisfying sweetness as well as beneficial nutrients, but limit fruit consumption to two or three pieces per day—more than that can raise triglyceride levels unless you are extremely active.

2. **Avoid health-damaging fats.** Although the trend in recent years has been toward low-fat diets, fat is not an optional nutrient—it is essential for your health. However, it *is* true that eating the

wrong types of fats damages cells, is a primary contributing factor to cancer and heart disease, and speeds up the aging process. On the other hand, eating healthful fats protects you against cancer, heart disease, and other degenerative diseases and helps to keep you young.

Fat is necessary for the absorption of fat-soluble vitamins such as vitamins A, E, D, K, beta-carotene, and CoQ-10 and is necessary for the creation of cell membranes. Fat also helps to balance blood-sugar levels by slowing the release of glucose into the bloodstream and is necessary for the production of prostaglandins, powerful hormone-like substances that play a role in many vital functions of the body including hormonal balance and proper immune function.

Unhealthful fats you should avoid include polyunsaturated oils, hydrogenated oils, and saturated fats. Polyunsaturated oils such as safflower, corn, soybean, and sunflower oils are extremely detrimental to your health. They quickly oxidize, turning rancid and creating free radicals, which injure healthy cells. Polyunsaturated oils become even more toxic when they undergo the process of hydrogenation to become margarine or shortening. Hydrogenation creates transfatty acids, an unnatural and dangerous fat that impairs healthy cell function, clogs arteries, lowers beneficial HDL cholesterol, depresses the immune system, and stimulates the growth of cancer cells. Not only are hydrogenated and partially hydrogenated fats sources of harmful free radicals, but once inside your body, they continue to oxidize and to create more free radicals. Many processed foods contain transfatty acids—you can identify them by the ingredients hydrogenated or partially hydrogenated oils on food labels. In addition to eliminating polyunsaturated and hydrogenated oils, also cut down on saturated fats, found primarily in red meat, whole-milk dairy products, poultry skin, and palm and coconut oils. These fats can raise cholesterol levels and increase the risk of cardiovascular disease.

The healthiest form of fat to use in your kitchen is extra-virgin olive oil. Olive oil is a monounsaturated fat and slow to oxidize. In addition, it offers a variety of health-protective benefits, such as decreasing levels of harmful LDL cholesterol and increasing levels of beneficial HDL cholesterol. It also makes cell membranes more resistant to the destructive effects of free radicals and helps to prevent heart disease and cancer. Peanut and canola oils are also monounsaturated fats, but peanut oil is often contaminated with pesticide residues and contains naturally occurring toxins. Canola oil, made from rapeseed, is also likely to be contaminated with pesticides and is extracted with toxic solvents if it is conventionally produced. Organic expeller-pressed canola oil is available, and some people like it because it is virtually flavorless. However, it does not have the health-protective benefits of olive oil.

3. Eat sufficient amounts of essential fatty acids. Essential fatty acids are special types of fats that are the building blocks of prostaglandins, the hormone-like substances that regulate virtually every important physiological process in the body. Prostaglandins play critical roles in cardiovascular, immune, and reproductive functions and also influence the nervous system. Because your body cannot manufacture essential fatty acids, you must obtain them through a diet that contains sufficient and balanced amounts of both omega-3 and omega-6 fatty acids. The ideal ratio of omega-6 to omega-3 fatty acids is about three to one, but the average American diet contains up to 25 times as many omega-6 fats as omega-3s. This imbalance is largely caused by food-processing methods that destroy omega-3 fatty acids, and also because omega-6 fats are prevalent in commonly eaten foods such as vegetable oils, meats, eggs, and grains. Omega-3 oils are not found in nearly as many foods; the best sources are cold-water fish such as salmon, mackerel, herring, sardines, and tuna, and some vegetable foods such as walnuts, and flaxseeds.

Omega-3 oils protect the cardiovascular system by raising levels of beneficial HDL cholesterol and lowering triglycerides and blood pressure. They also help to prevent degenerative diseases such as cancer, diabetes, and arthritis, and skin diseases such as eczema and psoriasis. To provide your body with all the benefits of omega-3 fats, eat two or three servings of cold-water fish weekly, and take one tablespoon of flaxseed oil or one to two tablespoons of freshly ground flaxseeds daily.

4. Eat plenty of high-fiber foods. A high-fiber diet is essential for preventing constipation as well as degenerative diseases such as cancer, heart disease, and varicose veins. Fiber speeds up the movement of wastes through the intestinal tract, which helps to cleanse the body of toxic chemicals such as pesticides and also aids in the elimination of excess estrogen and cholesterol. The longer wastes remain in the body, the more opportunity there is for toxins to be reabsorbed into the bloodstream through the porous walls of the intestines.

There are basically two types of fiber: insoluble and soluble. Insoluble fiber is the indigestible part of plants, such as the outer husk of wheat. This type of fiber creates bulk and stimulates the intestinal contractions that move wastes out of the body. Soluble fiber dissolves in water and forms a gel-like substance in the intestinal tract. Barley, oats, and legumes are rich in soluble fiber. This type of fiber absorbs toxic substances in the intestines, reduces harmful cholesterol, and helps to control bacterial toxins in the large intestine. Most plants contain a mixture of both types of fiber. For optimal health, eat a variety of whole grains, legumes, vegetables, and fruits to obtain all of the health benefits of different fibers.

Legumes such as soybeans, black beans, lentils, and kidney beans have other health-protective benefits in addition to being high in soluble fiber. Because they are digested slowly, they help to stabilize blood-sugar levels. They also contain substances called protease inhibitors, natural enzymes that inhibit carcinogens in the intestinal tract. Add beans to salads, include them in soups, and use them in sandwich spreads and dips. Many people initially have difficulty digesting beans because the complex sugars they contain require specific digestive enzymes. Eating beans frequently will help your body develop the enzymes needed to digest them easily. Begin with small amounts to give your digestive system an opportunity to adjust, and be sure to cook beans properly. You can eliminate most of the problematic sugars with the following method: Soak dried beans for at least four hours and preferably overnight. Pour off the soaking water, rinse, and add fresh water. Bring to a boil, and simmer until thoroughly tender. Adding fresh ginger root or fennel seed also helps to make beans more digestible.

5. Eat soy foods often. Soy foods are excellent sources of vegetable protein and are loaded with protective compounds that help to protect cells from free-radical damage. They contain powerful natural chemicals called isoflavones, plant hormones that ease menopausal symptoms and help to prevent osteoporosis and reproductive cancers. Soybeans also help to cleanse the arteries by increasing levels of beneficial HDL cholesterol and blocking the harmful effects of LDL cholesterol. For optimal protection, eat soy daily in the form of four ounces of tofu or tempeh, one cup of soy milk, or one-half cup of cooked soybeans. As with other beans, you may want to add soy gradually to your diet to give your intestinal tract an opportunity to adjust.

6. Eat calcium-rich foods. To help maintain bone strength and to keep your cardiovascular and nervous systems healthy, eat calcium-rich foods daily. Dairy products are high in calcium, but many women have difficulty digesting them. Fermented milk products such as yogurt or goat-milk products are often easier to digest. Don't rely solely on dairy products for calcium, but eat a wide variety of calcium-rich foods such as almonds, broccoli, collards, kale, legumes, oranges, sesame seeds, tofu, and sardines, and take calcium supplements for insurance.

7. Avoid excess sugar. The desire for the sweet taste is natural, and is an instinct that helped our early ancestors find sources of concentrated energy and avoid foods that might be poisonous. However, sugar is far out of balance in the modern diet, because sugar-laden desserts and snacks have become daily fare, and sweeteners are added to almost every processed food from salad dressings to juices. A high-sugar diet promotes the growth of unhealthful opportunistic microorganisms such as *Candida albicans* in the digestive tract and is a prime contributor to degenerative diseases such as diabetes and atherosclerosis. Sugar also knocks out your immune function—even one average serving of sugar hinders your immunity for several hours.

Sugar is detrimental to your health in all of its many guises, including sucrose, glucose, maltose, dextrose, corn syrup, and even sweeteners that are popularly thought to be healthful alternatives such as honey, molasses, and maple syrup. Ideally, eat sugar primarily as it occurs in whole foods, such as found in fresh fruits and sweet vegetables such as carrots, winter squashes, and sweet potatoes and reserve concentrated sweets for occasional treats. Make sure that you have adequate protein and fat in your diet, because they keep blood-sugar levels stable, which lessens the desire for sweets. If you eat sugar to boost your energy, try other more healthful ways of increasing your energy levels (see Chapter 12).

8. Avoid caffeine. Caffeine is a powerful stimulant drug that stresses your nervous system and contributes to insomnia and anxiety. By overstimulating the adrenal glands, it creates a state of chronic stress, resulting in fatigue after the initial stimulant effect wears off. Caffeine also has laxative and diuretic properties and can deplete nutrients such as calcium. Osteoporosis, PMS, and menopausal problems are all made worse by caffeine.

Caffeine is highly addictive, and giving it up often causes headaches, fatigue, and irritability for several days while your body detoxifies. Stick with eliminating it, and you'll feel like a new person within a few days. Coffee, black tea, chocolate, colas and other soft drinks, and many over-the-counter drugs including stimulants, cold remedies, and pain medications all contain caffeine. Green tea also contains a small amount of caffeine, but it generally does not cause the negative side effects of other sources of caffeine and has potent health-protective properties that make it a healthful beverage.

9. Drink plenty of water. Our bodies are approximately 60 percent water and require about two quarts of fluids daily to stay well-hydrated and maintain healthy organ function. Not drinking enough fluids causes toxins to build up in the body, and dehydration is a common cause of fatigue. About half of your need for fluids is provided in the foods you eat, especially if you eat plenty of vegetables and fruits. Pure spring water or filtered water is the best option for supplying the rest of the fluids your body needs. Get into the habit of drinking four to six glasses of water daily, preferably between meals.

Guidelines for a Health-Enhancing Diet

- Fresh vegetables: five or more servings daily (emphasize carotene-rich dark-leafy green and deep-yellow-orange vegetables and cruciferous vegetables such as broccoli, cabbage, and cauliflower)
- Fresh fruit: two to three servings daily (emphasize fruits rich in protective phytonutrients such as oranges, blueberries, strawberries, and mangoes)

- Complex carbohydrates: two or more servings daily (include one-half cup or more of legumes such as black beans, garbanzo beans, or lentils, which are good sources of soluble fiber and help to keep blood-sugar levels stable)
- Lean protein: two three-to-four ounce servings daily (eat cold-water fish such as salmon, sardines, and mackerel two to three times a week for omega-3 oils)
- Soy foods: one serving daily (one-half cup tempeh or tofu or one cup soy milk. Tofu or tempeh can fulfill one of your protein servings)
- Healthful fats: approximately 20–30 percent of your daily diet in the form of extra-virgin olive oil, raw nuts and seeds, and avocados
- Omega-3 essential fatty acids: several servings per week (found in cold-water fish, flaxseeds, pumpkin seeds, and walnuts)
- Calcium-rich foods: one to two servings of low-fat dairy products such as yogurt or goat cheese if you digest them well, or a couple of servings of other high-calcium foods such as dark-leafy greens, sardines, sesame seeds, and almonds along with a calcium supplement

Additional Health-Protective Foods:

- Pure water: four to six glasses daily
- Garlic: one clove or more daily to enhance immune function and protect against cardiovascular disease
- Shiitake mushrooms: six or more weekly to strengthen immune function and protect against cancer
- Green tea, three cups daily for its powerful antioxidant properties (can fulfill part of your water requirement)

How to Use Dietary Supplements

Even if you are eating an optimal diet, it is difficult to get enough of the antioxidants and other nutrients that help to protect your body against premature aging and degenerative diseases. Don't rely on supplements alone to build health, but do include them as part of a comprehensive approach to creating optimal energy, vitality, and longevity.

For best absorption of supplements, take capsules, which are more easily broken down and absorbed in the digestive tract than are tablets. Take supplements with meals, because food enhances absorption and lessens the possibility of stomach upset. Some nutrients, such as vitamin A, E, D, K, beta-carotene, and CoQ-10 are fat-soluble and must be taken with a meal that contains some fat in order to be properly assimilated. Just as with foods, supplements are best absorbed when you take them when you are relaxed, so avoid swallowing a handful of supplements while running out the door.

You can improve your absorption of supplements by strengthening your digestion. Taking an herbal digestive tonic before meals helps to stimulate the production of digestive fluids (see page 197 for a recipe for an herbal digestive tonic). Cultivating a healthy population of beneficial intestinal flora also enhances nutrient absorption. Eat yogurt daily that contains live beneficial bacteria such as *Lactobacillus acidophilus,* or take supplements of friendly flora such as acidophilus and bifidobacterium. Beneficial bacteria also help to protect against the overpopulation of problem-causing microorganisms such as *Candida albicans,* decrease the formation of free radicals in the intestinal tract, and are essential for healthy immune functioning.

Twelve Supplements for Optimal Health

1. High-potency mutivitamin-mineral. Choose a high-quality supplement that provides a wide range of all of the basic vitamins and minerals. Do not take a supplement that contains iron if you are postmenopausal—iron can accumulate to dangerous levels in the bloodstream and is implicated in cancer and heart disease.

2. Vitamin C. A powerful antioxidant, vitamin C enhances immune function, helps to prevent cancer and atherosclerosis, strengthens blood vessels, and blocks free-radical damage that can cause cataracts and macular degeneration. Take 1,000 to 2,000 milligrams daily in divided doses throughout the day to keep your cells continually saturated.

3. Vitamin E. By protecting cells against free-radical damage, vitamin E helps to prevent atherosclerosis, heart attacks, strokes, and cancer, and also strengthens immune function and helps to prevent mental deterioration caused by aging. Take 400 to 800 units daily in the form of d-alpha tocopherol or mixed tocopherols, and take with a meal that contains some fat for proper absorption. If you have high blood pressure, consult your doctor before taking large doses of vitamin E.

4. Beta-carotene. A potent antioxidant that works together with vitamins C and E to maintain a high level of cell protection, beta-carotene helps to prevent cancer and heart disease and enhances immune function. Beta-carotene is abundant in deep-yellow-orange fruits and vegetables and dark-leafy greens, but many health practitioners advise supplementing with 10,000 units of beta-carotene in the form of mixed carotenoids daily. For optimal health, eat a wide variety of beta-carotene-rich foods to obtain other nutrients that may have equally important health benefits.

5. B-complex vitamins. Look for a multivitamin that contains 50 to 100 milligrams per day of B-1, B-2, B-3, B-5, and B-6, plus at least 400 micrograms of folic acid, which is essential for preventing high levels of homocysteine in the blood, an amino acid that is strongly linked to atherosclerosis and heart disease. If you have high homocysteine levels or heart disease, you may need 1,000 micrograms or more of folic acid daily—consult your health practitioner for guidance.

B-complex vitamins, especially B-12, also help to prevent age-related mental deterioration. With age, B-12 absorption is often impaired, and what appears to be senile dementia, memory loss, or Alzheimer's disease may simply be caused by a deficiency of B-12. Supplements of B-12 are more easily absorbed than are food sources. If you show signs of deficiency, you may need more B-12 than is supplied in a multivitamin, up to 1,000 micrograms per day. Sublingual tablets or a nasal spray of B-12 are the most easily absorbable forms.

6. Selenium. A potent antioxidant, selenium is an essential building block for the body's own powerful antioxidant glutathione. Selenium enhances immune function and helps to prevent cancer

and heart disease. Take 200 micrograms daily. Do not exceed the recommended dosage because in large doses selenium can be toxic.

7. Calcium. An essential mineral for keeping bones strong, calcium also calms the nervous system, helps to prevent high blood pressure, and improves immune function by strengthening cell membranes. Take 800 milligrams daily, or 1,200 milligrams if you do not eat many calcium-rich foods. Calcium citrate is the most easily absorbed form—for best assimilation, divide into two or three doses and take with meals.

8. Magnesium. As important as calcium for maintaining bone strength, magnesium also lowers blood pressure, calms the nervous system, and prevents irregular heart rhythm (arrhythmias). Magnesium also blocks free-radical damage, enhances immunity, and by balancing blood-sugar levels helps to prevent diabetes. Take 400 to 600 milligrams daily in the form of citrate, malate, aspartate, gluconate, or lactate. Avoid taking more than 600 milligrams daily because excessive magnesium can cause diarrhea.

9. Zinc. Essential for proper immune functioning, zinc helps to rejuvenate the thymus gland, which commonly shrinks with age and is an essential component of the immune system. Zinc also has antioxidant properties. Take 15 to 30 milligrams daily, and be sure that the multivitamin supplement you are taking also includes copper, which can be depleted by excess zinc. Do not exceed the recommended dosage of zinc because too much can suppress immune functioning.

10. Chromium. By helping to decrease insulin and blood-sugar levels, chromium aids in preventing diabetes and atherosclerosis and the accelerated aging of tissues caused by high-insulin levels. Take 200 micrograms daily.

11. CoEnzyme Q-10. A potent antioxidant vitamin that is essential for maintaining a healthy cardiovascular system, CoQ-10 strengthens heart function, protects the arteries, and lowers blood pressure. It also enhances immune function and plays a critical role in the energy production within cells. Take 30 to 100 milligrams daily, preferably at breakfast and with a small amount of fat to increase absorption.

12. Grapeseed extract. With approximately 50 times the antioxidant potency of either vitamin C or vitamin E, grapeseed extract is a powerful protector of cell health. It contains compounds called proanthocyanidins that reduce the risk of degenerative diseases and help to slow the aging process. Take an extract that provides approximately 150 milligrams daily.

Chapter 27

Natural Beauty at Midlife and Beyond

Because changes in outward appearance are more readily apparent than changes in internal organs, these are most likely the first signs of growing older that a woman notices. It's not uncommon for women to feel a sense of loss associated with physical changes. But it is essential to recognize that true beauty at any age emanates from a woman's vitality and her involvement in life. It's important to honor the process of aging and to regard with love the lines on your face and the gray hairs that pay tribute to the years of life experience you have. At the same time, many of the physical changes that we associate with aging are exacerbated by years of accumulated neglect, including lack of essential nutrients, insufficient exercise, not enough sleep, and too much stress. The more attention that you pay to eating a healthful diet, exercising, getting enough rest, and reducing stress in your life, the better you will look and feel.

At midlife, it's more important than ever to nurture your body with exquisite care. Making positive changes in the way you care for yourself shows up as increased beauty, because your outward appearance is a barometer of your health and emotional well-being. To look your best, concentrate on creating beauty from the inside out.

Creating a Healthy Foundation for Beauty

To create a healthy internal environment that will enhance your unique beauty, make sure that you are eating a diet that supplies your body with optimal levels of all the nutrients it needs for healthy skin, hair, and nails. For specific guidelines for a health-and-beauty-enhancing diet, see Chapter 26.

Essential fatty acids in the form of omega-6 and omega-3 fats are particularly important for healthy skin and hair. Deficiencies are common, especially of omega-3 fatty acids, and often manifest as dry skin, brittle hair, or hair loss. Take one tablespoon of flaxseed oil (a rich source of omega-3 fatty acids) daily, or two tablespoons for one month or more if your skin and hair are very dry. Once your skin and hair have become softer, reduce the amount of flaxseed oil you are taking to one tablespoon per day. Gamma linolenic acid (GLA) is another essential fatty acid that is critical for healthy skin and hair. GLA is made by the body in small amounts, but is often lacking because production decreases with age. Taking supplemental GLA can result in profound differences in skin and hair health. Take 240 milligrams of GLA daily in the form of evening primrose oil, black currant oil, or borage oil.

All antioxidant vitamins and minerals enhance beauty, especially the appearance of the skin, by preventing free-radical damage. The destructive effects of free radicals are thought to be a primary cause of aging—for example, wrinkling and sagging skin is largely caused by free-radical damage triggered by excessive exposure to the ultraviolet rays of the sun. Taking optimal amounts of a variety of antioxidants helps to block the damaging effects of free radicals (see Chapter 26 for guidelines for supplements).

Keeping all your organs of detoxification working efficiently also helps to keep you looking your best. Your skin is part of your detoxification system, and if your intestines, liver, or kidneys are overburdened with toxins, your skin will suffer. You can keep your intestines healthy by eating a high-fiber diet and taking beneficial flora supplements (such as *Lactobacillus acidophilus*) when needed to replenish friendly intestinal bacteria. Your liver will function optimally if you avoid toxic substances and take herbs such as *milk thistle* to enhance your liver function. And your kidneys will work most efficiently if you drink plenty of pure water to aid them in their role of flushing toxic substances out of your body. For more information on supporting your organs of detoxification, see Chapter 12.

Maintaining Youthful Skin

Like your other body organs, your skin begins to slow down its functions as you age. As levels of estrogen and progesterone decline, skin becomes drier, thinner, and secretes less oil. Circulation decreases, and wrinkles appear when collagen and elastin, proteins in the skin that provide elasticity, break down. The rate of cell production and turnover decreases, and cells grow thicker and more tightly packed together. Common signs of aging skin include unevenness of skin texture and pigmentation, wrinkles, and "age spots," the brown patches caused by accumulated sun damage that appear on the face, chest, and the backs of the hands.

However, most of the skin changes that are blamed on aging are primarily the result of long-term exposure to the sun's ultraviolet rays. Compare the skin on the underside of your arm (which rarely is bared to the sun) to the skin on your face. If your facial skin had never been exposed to the sun, it would probably not look much different at age 50 than it did at when you were 20. Sun damages not only the top layer of skin, but the underlying supportive layer of collagen and elastin as well, which causes wrinkling and sagging.

Fortunately, it's never too late to begin improving the condition of your skin because skin cells have the ability to repair at least some of the damage caused by the sun's ultraviolet rays. Studies show that women who use a sunscreen daily experience significant improvement in the condition of their skin after only six months. Obviously, the degree of improvement is related to how much sun damage you have incurred, but the important point is that avoiding further sun exposure will help you have better-looking skin. Use a sunscreen with an SPF (sun protection factor) of 15 or higher every day, even during the winter and on cloudy days, and make sure that the sunscreen you are using blocks out both UVA and UVB rays. While using an SPF 15 sunscreen allows you to stay out in the sun 15 times longer than you normally would be able to without burning, the best way to prevent sun damage is to avoid direct sun exposure when the sun's rays are the strongest, which is usually between the hours of 10 A.M. and 3 P.M. If you are outdoors during those hours, make an effort to stay in the shade as much as possible, and use physical barriers such as tightly woven long-sleeved clothing, sunglasses, and a broad-brimmed hat.

Moisture: The Key to Beautiful Skin

Many women find that their skin becomes drier after the age of 35. This may be a welcome change for those who suffered from oily skin earlier in life, but women with normal or dry skin may find that their skin appears flaky, tight, and lacks the lustrous appearance that moisture imparts. Skin dryness is caused not only by moisture loss from the skin's outer layer, but also from a lack of moisture moving upward from the underlying layers of the skin. Applying a moisturizer softens and moisturizes the top layer of skin, but the effects are only temporary.

To have soft, pliable, moist skin, you need to lubricate your skin from the inside. Drink at least six glasses of pure water daily and eat plenty of fresh vegetables and fruits to keep your body tissues well-hydrated. Don't wait to drink until you are thirsty because by then you are already dehydrated. Instead, keep a container of water handy for sipping throughout the day. If you find plain water boring, try making unsweetened or lightly sweetened herbal teas such as linden flower, chamomile, or mint.

A moist external environment also provides moisture for your skin and helps to keep cells plump. Use a humidifier during the winter months to counteract the drying effects of indoor heating and also during the summer if you use air conditioning or if you live in a dry climate. Misting your skin frequently with pure mineral water or a facial mist containing floral waters and aromatherapy essential oils provides an immediate and refreshing boost of moisture for your skin throughout the day. (See the suggestions on page 287 for making a variety of facial mists.) Soaking in a warm bath is an effective way of hydrating the skin of your entire body. Avoid excessively hot water, because it can remove protective oils from your skin. After a 15-minute soak, massage your body with an aromatherapy oil (see suggestions on page 295) while you are still wet from the bath, and then gently pat your skin dry with a towel. The thin layer of aromatherapy oil acts as a protective barrier that prevents the evaporation of moisture that your skin has absorbed from the bath.

Exfoliate to Speed Up Skin Renewal

Your skin naturally sheds dead cells every day, which helps to keep it smooth and fresh looking. But after the age of 35, the dead cells that make up the outer layer of your skin are not shed as rapidly as when you were younger. As dead cells accumulate, they make your skin look dull and dry and you lose the healthy, radiant look that characterizes youthful skin. You can greatly improve the appearance of your skin by regularly removing the top layer of dead skin cells, a process called exfoliation. Exfoliation is accomplished by using grainy scrubs that physically remove dead cells through gentle abrasion, or fruit-enzyme skin peels or alpha-hydroxy acid skin peels, which dissolve the top layer of dead skin cells.

Natural scrubs are made from finely ground fibrous plant material such as oatmeal, corn meal, almonds, and apricot kernels. Be cautious when using grainy scrubs, because many are too harsh to use on the delicate skin of your face. For a gentle scrub that will not irritate your skin, try the recipe on page 283. Although many grainy scrubs are too abrasive to use on your face, they are perfect to use as an allover exfoliator for your body. Your body builds up dead skin cells just as your face does and benefits from a weekly exfoliating treatment. Try the recipe on page 294 if you want to make your own body scrub.

Fruit-enzyme peels are made from fruit or vegetable enzymes that exfoliate the skin in approximately 20 minutes without scrubbing. Many contain green papaya, which contains the protein-digesting enzyme papain. Dead skin cells are composed primarily of protein, and enzyme peels digest the dead skin cells on the surface of the skin without harming new cell growth. Enzyme peels are gentle exfoliators and leave skin noticeably smoother and softer after only one treatment. They can be used as part of a weekly or monthly facial treatment and can even be used daily as part of a program to rejuvenate aging skin. For a mild, natural enzyme peel, try the recipe on page 285.

Alpha-hydroxy acids are natural exfoliators derived from foods such as citrus fruits (citric acid), sour milk (lactic acid), grapes (tartaric acid), sugar cane (glycolic acid), and apples (malic acid). These gentle, natural acids work by loosening the "glue" that binds the outermost layer of surface cells together, which increases the shedding of dead skin cells and encourages the formation of new skin cells. The idea of using the natural acids found in foods to renew the skin is not new—Cleopatra bathed in buttermilk, and red wine has been used for centuries as a skin wash. Alpha-hydroxy acids improve skin texture and color, reduce fine lines and age spots, and make pores appear smaller. Although you will usually notice smoother skin after the first treatment, you'll need to use alpha-hydroxy acids on a regular basis for two months or longer to see a significant improvement in skin texture and diminishment of fine lines. There are a variety of natural products available, and most contain between 5 and 15 percent alpha-hydroxy acids. Products that contain higher percentages of alpha-hydroxy acids will create faster results, but often cause stinging or tingling sensations when applied to the skin. These reactions are not usually a cause for concern, but severe stinging or redness indicates an undue sensitivity or allergic reaction and you should try a different product with a lower concentration of alpha-hydroxy acids. You can also make your own facial masks based on yogurt and fruits rich in alpha-hydroxy acids with the recipes on pages 284–86.

Basic Principles for Healthy Hair

Your hair is actually an extension of your skin, and like your skin, is a direct reflection of your internal health. While topical treatments such as conditioners can smooth the surface of your hair and make it appear softer, true hair health begins deep beneath the surface in the hair follicles. A nutrient-rich diet is essential for creating strong, healthy hair. Stringent dieting and food plans that overly restrict fat and protein intake can cause dull, dry, and thinning hair. Follow the guidelines for a health-enhancing diet in Chapter 26, and make sure to eat enough protein (at least two three-ounce servings every day) and plenty of essential fatty acids (one tablespoon of flax oil and 240 milligrams of GLA supplements daily). Essential fatty acids are crucial for keeping your hair strong, pliable, and shiny. But even if you are eating a healthful diet, poor digestion and assimilation can wreak havoc with your hair, skin, and nails. To improve your digestion, take an herbal-digestive tonic daily, and see the other suggestions for optimizing your digestion in Chapter 20.

Women who experience thinning hair at midlife and beyond often have hormonal imbalances associated with the adrenal glands, thyroid, and reproductive organs. Take the hormone-balancing tonic on page 86, and also support your adrenal glands by eliminating sugar and caffeine and using an adrenal tonic herb such as *Siberian ginseng*. (For more suggestions for improving adrenal health, refer to Chapter 12.) The Chinese herb *Ho shou wu* is also an excellent tonic to take if you are experiencing hair loss. It strengthens thyroid function, is a gentle energy-building herb, and enhances hair growth.

Good circulation is essential for healthy hair. Daily aerobic exercise stimulates circulation throughout the body, and inverted yoga postures such as the shoulder stand are especially helpful for increasing circulation to the scalp. In addition, yoga relieves emotional stress, which plays a role in hormonal imbalances and consequent hair loss. Massaging your scalp daily with a blend of essential oils especially formulated to stimulate the hair follicles can also help to restore scalp and hair health (see recipe on page 290).

Herbal Skin and Hair Care

Herbs have been used for centuries to cleanse, moisturize, heal, and beautify the skin and hair. Early Egyptians protected themselves against the ravages of the sun and aging by anointing their bodies with oils infused with rose petals and myrrh. In ancient Rome, the renowned physician Galen blended olive oil, beeswax, herbal extracts, and water to create the first skin cream. His recipe still

forms the basis for moisturizers made today. Herbs have traditionally been combined with other natural ingredients such as honey,
oats, almond oil and fragrant essential oils to soften and soothe dry
or irritated skin, stimulate circulation and cell regeneration, and
eliminate toxins and the blemishes they cause.

For optimal skin and hair health—as well as your overall well-
being—avoid body-care products that contain synthetic chemicals.
In this century, mass-market-oriented cosmetics manufacturers have
replaced natural substances with less expensive synthetic ingredients. Instead of delicate almond oil, for example, a conventional
moisturizer is likely to contain mineral oil, a petroleum by-product
that clogs pores. Soothing skin toners such as rosewater and witch
hazel have been replaced with harsh chemicals such as acetone—
the active ingredient in nail-polish remover. In fact, a wide range of
well-known cancer-causing chemicals such as formaldehyde and
talc are routinely used in commercial cosmetics. Not only can these
chemicals cause dryness, irritation, and allergic reactions, but your
skin (including your scalp) is more than just a covering for your
body—it is, in fact, your largest organ and readily absorbs about 60
percent of any substance that is applied to it. The most healthful and
prudent approach is to choose your body-care products as carefully as you choose the foods you eat.

There are many healthful natural body-care products available at
natural products stores and by mail order. You can also easily create
your own herbal skin and body-care products in the same way that
cosmetics have been made for centuries with the following simple
recipes.

Skin-Care Formulas

Choose from the following herbs and essential oils when making
skin-care products to customize the formulas to your needs.

DRY SKIN

Herbs: chamomile, comfrey, elder flower, rose
Essential oils: chamomile, sandalwood, rose

OILY SKIN

Herbs: lavender, peppermint, rosemary, yarrow

Essential oils: cypress, cedarwood, lavender

NORMAL SKIN

Herbs: calendula, chamomile, lavender, rose

Essential oils: lavender, geranium, rose

MATURE SKIN

Herbs: chamomile, comfrey, lavender, rose, rosemary

Essential oils: frankincense, lavender, rosemary, rose

SENSITIVE SKIN

Herbs: calendula, chamomile, comfrey, rose

Essential oils: chamomile, lavender, rose

Herbal Facial Sauna

An herbal facial sauna gently deep cleanses your skin. Warm herbal steam opens the pores, washes away impurities, and also helps to hydrate the skin.

> *1–1/2 quarts water*
>
> *6 tablespoons herbal mixture for your skin type (see page 280)*
>
> *Almond or jojoba oil (optional)*

1. Bring water to boil in a large pot.
2. Turn off the heat, add herbal mixture, cover the pot, and allow the herbs to steep for 5 minutes.
3. Wash your face with a gentle cleanser and warm water. If your skin is dry, apply a thin layer of almond or jojoba oil to your face.

4. Place the pot on a table, remove the lid, and make a towel tent over your head and the pot to capture the steam. Stay under the towel for 10 minutes to allow the steam to cleanse your pores. Lift the towel as necessary to regulate the temperature, and take care to not burn yourself with the steam.

5. Rinse with tepid water, and follow with a gentle facial scrub and a facial mask if desired.

Aromatherapy Facial Sauna

This is a simplified version of an herbal facial sauna. Essential oils have a wonderful fragrance and are beneficial for your skin.

> *1–1/2 quarts water*
>
> *3 drops essential oil appropriate for your skin type (see page 280)*

1. Pour boiling water into a large, heatproof bowl. Add essential oil.

2. Make a towel tent over your head and the bowl with a large towel to capture the steam. Lift the towel as necessary to regulate the temperature, and take care to not burn yourself with the steam. Stay under the towel for 10 minutes to allow the steam to cleanse your pores.

3. Rinse your face with tepid water, and follow with a gentle facial scrub and a facial mask if desired.

Lavender Facial Compress

This quick and fragrant facial compress is like a minisauna. It's simple enough to be used as part of your regular cleansing routine.

> *basin of warm water*
>
> *2 drops lavender essential oil*

1. Add lavender essential oil to a basin of very warm water.

2. Soak a washcloth in the scented water, wring out the cloth, and gently compress your face and neck with the cloth. Repeat several times, wringing out the cloth each time in the warm water.

Herbal Cleansing Milk

Milky cleansers are much gentler for your skin than soaps. Making your own herbal cleansing milk is easy. It will stay fresh for one week in the refrigerator. For longer storage, freeze in ice-cube trays and thaw out a cube as needed.

2 tablespoons calendula flowers

1 tablespoon chamomile flowers

1 tablespoon rose petals

1 cup whole milk

1. Combine calendula, chamomile, and rose petals with milk in a pint-size glass jar. Cover, and steep overnight in the refrigerator.
2. Strain through cheesecloth, rebottle, and store in the refrigerator.
3. To use, dampen your face with warm water and apply cleansing milk with a soft cosmetic sponge. Rinse well with warm water.

Gentle Cleansing Grains

These cleansing grains gently exfoliate the top layer of dead skin cells, leaving your skin silky smooth. They also make an excellent base for facial masks.

2 cups rolled oats

1/2 cup almonds

2 tablespoons dried rose petals

2 tablespoons dried lavender flowers

1. In a clean coffee grinder, finely grind the oats, almonds, and herbs in separate batches. Mix well, and store in a covered container in a cool, dry place.
2. To use, mix 1 heaping teaspoon of cleansing grains with enough warm water to make a creamy paste. If your skin is dry, add 1/2 teaspoon almond oil.
3. Gently massage the mixture into your skin and rinse well with warm water.
4. Follow with a toner and moisturizer.

Aromatherapy Facial Mask

This simple mask combines the purifying benefits of clay with fragrant essential oils. The addition of almond or jojoba oil keeps the
mask from drying your skin.

> *1/2 teaspoon cosmetic clay*
>
> *2 teaspoons plain yogurt*
>
> *1/2 teaspoon almond or jojoba oil*
>
> *2 drops essential oil appropriate for your skin type (see page 280)*

1. Combine cosmetic clay with yogurt, almond or jojoba oil, and
   essential oil of your choice.
2. Wash your face with warm water or use a *Lavender Facial
   Compress* (see page 282). Apply the mask.
3. After 15 minutes, remove the mask with a warm, wet washcloth and rinse thoroughly with warm water.
4. Follow with a toner and moisturizer.

Strawberry Exfoliating Mask

Strawberries, yogurt, and rosemary essential oil all have gentle exfoliating properties. Use this wonderfully fragrant mask when your
skin needs an invigorating boost.

> *1 medium strawberry*
>
> *1 teaspoon plain whole-milk yogurt*
>
> *1 teaspoon* Gentle Cleansing Grains
>
> *2 drops rosemary essential oil*

1. Thoroughly mash strawberry and blend with yogurt. Add rosemary essential oil and 1 teaspoon or more of *Gentle Cleansing
   Grains* (page 283) to make a spreadable mask.
2. Wash face with warm water or apply *Lavender Facial Compress*
   (page 282), and spread mask onto clean, damp skin.
3. After 15 minutes, remove with a warm, wet washcloth and
   rinse thoroughly with lukewarm water.
4. Follow with a toner and moisturizer.

Avocado Moisturizing Mask

This rich avocado mask can be used weekly as a treat to nourish dry skin.

> *1 tablespoon ripe avocado*
> *1 teaspoon plain whole-milk yogurt*
> *1 teaspoon* Gentle Cleansing Grains *(page 283) or cosmetic clay*
> *3 drops sandalwood essential oil*

1. Mash avocado and yogurt together until creamy.
2. Mix in *Gentle Cleansing Grains* or cosmetic clay and sandalwood oil to make a thick, spreadable mask.
3. Wash face with warm water or use *Lavender Facial Compress* (page 282) and apply mask to skin.
4. After 15 minutes, remove mask with a warm, wet washcloth and rinse thoroughly with lukewarm water.
5. Apply a toner and moisturizer.

Papaya Refining Mask

Papaya contains natural enzymes that exfoliate the top layer of dead skin cells, revealing soft and healthy skin beneath. Frankincense has cell-renewing properties.

> *1/4 cup diced papaya*
> *1 teaspoon honey*
> *2 drops frankincense essential oil*

1. Mash papaya with honey until thoroughly blended.
2. Add frankincense essential oil and mix well.
3. Apply *Lavender Facial Compress* (page 282) or wash your face with warm water, and apply mask. This mask tends to be runny, so protect your clothing with a towel and lie down and relax after applying the mask.
4. After 15 minutes, remove the mask with a warm, wet washcloth and rinse your face thoroughly with lukewarm water.
5. Apply a toner and moisturizer.

Fruit Enzyme Peel

The natural alpha-hydroxy acids in apples, strawberries, yogurt, and honey help to slough off dead skin cells. Chamomile provides soothing and healing properties.

> *1/4 cup diced apple*
>
> *2 strawberries, sliced*
>
> *1 tablespoon whole milk yogurt*
>
> *1 teaspoon honey*
>
> *2 teaspoons cosmetic clay (or more)*
>
> *2 drops chamomile essential oil*

1. Blend apple, yogurt, strawberries, and honey in blender until smooth.
2. Mix in chamomile essential oil and enough cosmetic clay to make a thin, spreadable mask.
3. Wash face, neck, and chest with warm water or apply *Lavender Facial Compress* (page 282).
4. Spread mask onto face, neck, and chest. Relax for 15 to 30 minutes.
5. Remove mask with a warm washcloth, and rinse well with warm water.
6. Apply a toner and moisturizer.

Herbal Facial Toner

Use this soothing herbal toner after washing your face to remove remaining traces of cleanser. It's also great as a skin refresher after exercising.

> *1 cup distilled witch hazel*
>
> *1 teaspoon each: dried chamomile, calendula, comfrey, elder flowers, and rose petals*
>
> *1 tablespoon vegetable glycerin*

1. Combine herbs and witch hazel in a glass jar with a tight-fitting lid. Allow the mixture to steep in a warm, dark place for two weeks.

2. After 2 weeks, strain the herbal mixture through several layers of cheesecloth or a coffee filter, reserving the liquid.

3. Add 1 tablespoon of vegetable glycerin, pour into a glass bottle, and shake to blend. Shake well before using.

4. To use, apply approximately 1 teaspoon to a cotton cosmetic square and gently cleanse your face and throat.

Aromatherapy Facial Mist

Use this fragrant facial mist to refresh and hydrate your skin throughout the day. Use the essential oils recommended here, or choose other essential oils appropriate for your skin type from the suggestions on page 280. Keep the total amount of essential oil to 30 drops or less.

1 tablespoon distilled witch hazel

20 drops lavender essential oil

10 drops rose or sandalwood essential oil

filtered water

1. Combine witch hazel and essential oils in a 6-ounce glass spray bottle.

2. Shake vigorously, and fill the bottle with filtered water.

3. Shake well before using.

Aloe-Lavender Facial Mist

Aloe vera, lavender, and frankincense all have cell-renewing properties and make a wonderfully fragrant facial mist.

6 ounces aloe vera juice

20 drops lavender essential oil

10 drops frankincense essential oil

1. Combine aloe vera juice with lavender and frankincense essential oils in a 6-ounce glass spray bottle. Shake vigorously.
2. Shake well before each use and mist skin as desired.

Herbal Eye Freshener

Chamomile, rose petals, and elder flowers soothe tired eyes and help to relieve puffiness.

1 tablespoon chamomile flowers

1 tablespoon rose petals

1 tablespoon elder flowers

2 cups water

1. Pour 2 cups boiling water over chamomile, rose petals, and elder flowers. Cover, and let steep until cool. Strain through several layers of cheesecloth, and chill in refrigerator.
2. Soak a clean washcloth in the herbal mixture and wring it out slightly.
3. Lie down, and place the washcloth over your closed eyes. Relax for 10 minutes.

Aromatherapy Facial Oil

Pure jojoba oil is an excellent facial moisturizer. Because it is similar to the skin's natural oils, it is easily absorbed. Fragrant essential oils add healing and rejuvenating properties.

1 ounce jojoba oil

10 drops of essential oil appropriate for your skin type (see page 280)

1. Combine essential oil (or a combination of essential oils) appropriate for your skin type with jojoba oil in a dark-glass bottle. A glass pharmacy bottle with a dropper works well for dispensing drops of oil.
2. After cleansing your skin with warm water, gently massage 3 to 4 drops of the moisturizing oil onto your damp skin with your fingertips.

Rich Aromatherapy Skin Cream

This wonderfully rich cream is excellent as a moisturizer for dry skin anywhere on your body.

> *1/4 cup almond oil*
>
> *2 tablespoons jojoba oil*
>
> *1 tablespoon vitamin-E oil*
>
> *2 tablespoons grated beeswax*
>
> *3 tablespoons rosewater*
>
> *10 drops lavender essential oil*
>
> *10 drops sandalwood essential oil*

1. Combine almond oil, jojoba oil, vitamin E, and beeswax in a small, heavy pot, and heat over low heat until beeswax melts.

2. Remove from heat, and cool to room temperature. The mixture will thicken slightly as it cools. Mix essential oils into the oil mixture after it has cooled.

3. Pour rose water into a blender, turn the blender on medium speed, and add the cooled oil slowly, blending until the mixture becomes thick and creamy.

4. Spoon the mixture into a glass jar and store in a cool, dark place.

How to Perform a Complete Facial:

1. Relax by applying a warm scented washcloth to your face (try the *Lavender Facial Compress* on page 282).

2. Cleanse your skin with *Herbal Cleansing Milk* (page 283) or your favorite mild cleanser. Apply the cleanser with gentle circular motions, and wipe it off with a warm, wet washcloth.

3. To deep cleanse skin, use an *Herbal Facial Sauna* (page 281) or *Aromatherapy Facial Sauna* (page 282).

4. Exfoliate your skin with *Gentle Cleansing Grains* (page 283) or apply the *Strawberry Exfoliating Mask* (page 284), *Papaya Refining Mask* (page 285), or *Fruit Enzyme Peel* (page 286), leaving the mask on your skin for 15 minutes. Relax, placing cotton pads soaked in *Herbal Eye Freshener* (page 288) onto your closed eyes.

5. Rinse your skin with warm water, and if you wish, apply a nourishing mask such as the *Avocado Moisturizing Mask* (page 285), and leave on your skin for 15 minutes.

6. Rinse your skin with warm water, gently pat dry, and apply the *Herbal Facial Toner* (page 286), *Aloe-Lavender Facial Mist* (page 287) or *Aromatherapy Facial Mist* (page 287).

7. Apply a small amount of *Aromatherapy Facial Oil* (page 288) or *Rich Aromatherapy Skin Cream* (page 289).

Hair-Care Formulas

Stimulating Scalp Treatment

The essential oils in this formula are traditionally used to stimulate hair growth. Apply this treatment to your scalp at least 1 hour before shampooing.

> *2 ounces jojoba oil*
>
> *15 drops rosemary essential oil*
>
> *10 drops lavender essential oil*
>
> *5 drops cedarwood essential oil*

1. Combine jojoba oil with rosemary, lavender, and cedarwood essential oils in a small dark-glass bottle. Shake well.

2. Apply 1/2 teaspoon or more to your scalp, massaging the oil into your scalp with your fingertips.

3. After 1 hour or longer (you can leave this scalp treatment on overnight) shampoo your hair as usual.

Deep-Conditioning Honey Hair Treatment

This deep conditioning treatment is beneficial for your hair and your scalp.

> *2 tablespoons jojoba oil*
>
> *2 teaspoons honey*

5 drops rosemary essential oil

5 drops sandalwood essential oil

1. Combine jojoba oil and honey in a small saucepan, and gently heat to a comfortably warm temperature. Add rosemary and sandalwood essential oils.

2. Dampen your hair and scalp with warm water.

3. Massage the warm oil mixture into your scalp with your fingertips, working the oil through your hair all the way to the ends.

4. Cover your hair with a shower cap and a hot, damp towel to help the oils penetrate more deeply. Leave in place for 30 minutes, replacing the hot towel as it cools.

5. Shampoo and follow with conditioner if necessary.

Aromatherapy Shampoo

You can customize unscented mild shampoos with herbal teas and essential oils especially suited to your hair and scalp type.

SHAMPOO FOR DRY HAIR

1/4 cup unscented mild, natural shampoo

1/4 cup strong calendula tea, cooled and strained

15 drops sandalwood essential oil

15 drops lavender essential oil

Combine all ingredients, and shake well before using.

SHAMPOO FOR OILY HAIR

1/4 cup unscented mild, natural shampoo

1/4 cup strong sage tea, cooled and strained

15 drops cedarwood essential oil

15 drops lavender essential oil

Combine all ingredients, and shake well before using.

Shampoo for normal hair

1/4 cup unscented mild natural shampoo
1/4 cup strong lavender tea, cooled and strained
20 drops lavender essential oil
10 drops rosemary or rose essential oil

Combine all ingredients and shake well before using.

Shampoo for problem scalps

1/4 cup unscented mild, natural shampoo
1/4 cup strong thyme tea, cooled and strained
10 drops eucalyptus essential oil
20 drops lavender essential oil

Combine all ingredients and shake well before using.

Shampoo for hair loss

1/4 cup unscented mild, natural shampoo
1/4 cup strong nettle tea, cooled and strained
20 drops rosemary essential oil
10 drops basil essential oil

Combine all ingredients and shake well before using.

Hand, Foot, and Nail Treatments

Herbal Foot Soak

Treat your feet to a little pampering with this softening and fragrant foot soak.

2 cups baking soda
1 teaspoon almond oil
5 drops lavender essential oil
5 drops sandalwood essential oil
handful dried or fresh rose petals

1. Fill a plastic tub large enough to comfortably hold both of your feet with hot water. Add baking soda and stir to dissolve.

2. Mix lavender and sandalwood essential oils with almond oil and add to the footbath. Float dried rose petals in the bath if you like.

3. Soak your feet for 10 minutes or longer to soften calluses and cuticles.

4. While your feet are still damp, gently remove calluses with a pumice stone or callus file. Push back your cuticles with an orangewood stick.

5. Apply *Aromatherapy Nail Oil* (page 294) to your toenails and cuticles, and massage a small amount of *Rich Aromatherapy Skin Cream* (page 289) into your feet.

Herbal Hand and Nail Soak

A warm herbal soak with fragrant essential oils softens your hands and makes it easy to shape up your nails and cuticles.

> *2 tablespoons calendula flowers*
> *2 tablespoons chamomile flowers*
> *1 teaspoon almond oil*
> *5 drops lavender essential oil*
> *5 drops frankincense essential oil*

1. Make a strong herbal tea by pouring 4 cups boiling water over calendula and chamomile flowers. Allow to steep until comfortably warm, and strain into a bowl large enough to hold both of your hands.

2. Add almond oil and lavender and frankincense essential oils.

3. Soak your hands in the warm bath for 10 minutes. Push back your cuticles with an orangewood stick while your hands are damp.

4. Pat your nails dry and massage a few drops of *Aromatherapy Nail Oil* (page 294) into your nails. Apply a small amount of *Rich Aromatherapy Skin Cream* (page 289) to your hands to seal in moisture.

Aromatherapy Nail Oil

This nail oil protects your nails from the brittleness and dryness caused by hot water, soaps, and nail-polish remover.

> *4 tablespoons jojoba oil*
>
> *10 drops sandalwood essential oil*
>
> *5 drops frankincense essential oil*

1. Combine jojoba oil with sandalwood and frankincense essential oils in a small dark glass bottle with a dropper. Shake well to thoroughly mix the oils.

2. Massage a few drops into nails and cuticles once a day, or more often if you wish.

Body Care and Baths

Skin-Renewing Body Scrub

This luxurious body scrub removes dull, dry skin and leaves skin silky smooth. It is gentle enough for all skin types, but use a light touch if you have sensitive skin, and do not apply to burned or irritated skin. Use a tub mat to avoid slipping in the shower.

> *1/4 cup uncooked rolled oats*
>
> *1/4 cup raw almonds*
>
> *1/4 cup corn flour or fine corn meal*
>
> *1 tablespoon almond oil or avocado oil*
>
> *5 drops lavender essential oil*
>
> *5 drops frankincense essential oil*

1. Grind the rolled oats and almonds in separate batches into a fine meal in a blender or coffee grinder. Place in a small plastic bowl.

2. Add corn flour, almond or avocado oil, and lavender and frankincense essential oils. Mix well.

3. Dampen your entire body in a warm shower. Using approximately 1 tablespoon at a time, massage the scrub into your skin, beginning with your calves and working your way up your body, including your neck, but avoiding your face.

4. Rinse well with warm water, and finish with a cool rinse.

Relaxing Mineral Bath

This bath combines minerals from the earth and sea for a concentrated mineral soak that will relax you while softening your skin.

> *2 cups baking soda*
> *1/2 cup Epsom salts*
> *1/2 cup sea salt*
> *5 drops lavender essential oil*
> *5 drops marjoram essential oil*

1. Fill your bathtub with comfortably warm water. Add the baking soda, Epsom salts, and sea salt to the tub while the water is running to dissolve the mineral salts.

2. Add the essential oils just before entering the tub, stirring the oils into the water with your hand.

3. Relax in the tub for 15 to 20 minutes and follow with a tepid shower.

Aromatherapy Body Oil

Smooth a few drops of this massage oil over your entire body immediately after emerging from a shower or bath while your skin is still damp. The oil seals moisture into your skin and creates a protective barrier against dryness.

> *2 ounces almond oil*
> *2 ounces jojoba oil*
> *10 drops lavender essential oil*
> *10 drops grapefruit essential oil*

10 drops frankincense essential oil

10 drops sandalwood essential oil

1. Combine all ingredients in a dark-glass bottle, and shake well. This oil goes a long way, especially if you are applying it to damp skin, so use only a small amount.

Silken Body Powder

Body dusting powders add a luxurious finishing touch to a bath. They give your skin a silky feel and absorb excess perspiration.

1 cup arrowroot powder

1/2 cup white cosmetic clay

1/2 cup dried rose petals

25 drops lavender essential oil

15 drops sandalwood essential oil

10 drops rose essential oil

1. Powder the rose petals in a clean coffee grinder.
2. Mix the arrowroot, clay, and powdered roses together in a nonporous bowl.
3. Add lavender, sandalwood, and rose essential oils and thoroughly mix the oil into the powder with your fingertips.
4. Store in a covered tin or glass jar to prevent the essential oils from dissipating, and allow the powder to mellow for a couple of days before using.
5. Apply with a powder puff or large soft brush, or package in a spice jar with a shaker top.

How to Cook for Health

Salads

Arugula with Avocado and Oranges

Arugula is a delicious, mildly bitter salad green with a nutty flavor. The bitter flavor stimulates digestive function. Serves 4.

> *1 bunch arugula*
>
> *1 head romaine*
>
> *1 medium cucumber, sliced in thin half-rounds*
>
> *1/4 small red onion, cut into paper-thin slices*
>
> *1 ripe avocado, sliced*
>
> *1 tablespoon extra-virgin olive oil*
>
> *1 tablespoon flaxseed oil*
>
> *1 teaspoon honey mustard*
>
> *1 teaspoon honey*
>
> *2 tablespoons freshly squeezed lemon juice*
>
> *2 tablespoons freshly squeezed orange juice*
>
> *1/8 teaspoon sea salt, or to taste*

1. Wash arugula and romaine, spin dry, and tear into large, bite-sized pieces. Add cucumber, red onion, and avocado.
2. Combine olive oil, flaxseed oil, mustard, and honey. Whisk in lemon and orange juice. Pour over salad and toss. Adjust seasonings and serve.

Warm Spinach Salad

Spinach is rich in vitamin K, and garlic and shiitake have powerful immune-enhancing properties. Serves 4.

> *1/2 cup thinly sliced purple onion*
>
> *1 cup fresh shiitake mushrooms, stemmed and sliced*
>
> *3 cloves garlic, minced*
>
> *2 tablespoons extra-virgin olive oil*
>
> *2/3 cup balsamic vinegar*
>
> *2 roasted red peppers, cut into thin strips*
>
> *2 pounds fresh spinach, washed and dried*
>
> *1/4 cup feta cheese*

1. In a medium skillet, sauté onion in olive oil for 2 minutes. Add shiitake and garlic and sauté for an additional 2 minutes.
2. Add balsamic vinegar, and lower heat. Simmer until mushrooms are tender, approximately 3 minutes.
3. Add roasted red pepper, cook for 1 minute, and remove from heat.
4. Pour over spinach and toss until spinach is completely coated with dressing.
5. Crumble feta cheese over salad and serve.

Cabbage Salad with Apples and Currants

This salad is rich in fiber and protective phytonutrients. Walnuts and flaxseed oil add essential fatty acids. Serves 4.

> *4 cups finely shredded purple cabbage*
> *1/4 cup dried currants*
> *2 scallions, finely minced*
> *2 tablespoons flaxseed oil*
> *2 tablespoons freshly squeezed lemon juice*
> *1/4 teaspoon sea salt*
> *1 crisp apple, diced*
> *1/4 cup walnuts, coarsely chopped*

1. Combine all ingredients except apple and walnuts and allow to stand for 1 hour or longer to allow cabbage to soften.
2. Add apple and walnuts just before serving and adjust seasonings.

Carrot-Apple Salad

Combining carrots and apples provides a double dose of pectin, the soluble fiber that cleanses arteries. Walnuts and flaxseed oil add health-enhancing omega-3 fatty acids. Serves 4.

> *3 cups grated carrots*
> *1 large, firm apple, diced*
> *2 tablespoons currants*
> *4 tablespoons walnuts, chopped coarsely*
> *1/2 cup freshly squeezed orange juice*
> *2 teaspoons freshly squeezed lemon juice*
> *1 tablespoon flaxseed oil*
> *1/2 teaspoon ground cinnamon*
> *pinch of sea salt*

1. Mix together grated carrots, apple, currants, and walnuts.
2. Combine orange juice, lemon juice, flaxseed oil, cinnamon, and sea salt. Pour over carrot combination, and mix well. Adjust seasonings to taste.

Avocado-Grapefruit Salad

Avocados and grapefruit are both rich sources of glutathione, a powerful antioxidant that neutralizes harmful free radicals. Serves 4.

1 large pink grapefruit

1 large ripe avocado

1 tablespoon extra-virgin olive oil

1 head butter lettuce

1/4 bunch tender arugula greens

sea salt and fresh ground black pepper

1. Peel and section the grapefruit. Cut the avocado in half and slice into 1-inch slices, then slice in half again. Gently combine the avocado and grapefruit.
2. Wash and dry the lettuce. Keep small leaves whole, and tear larger leaves into smaller pieces. Add the grapefruit and avocado and drizzle with olive oil. Season with sea salt and fresh-ground black pepper.

Broccoli and White Bean Salad

This bean-and-vegetable salad is exceptionally rich in soluble fibers. It makes a great lunch or summer supper. Serves 4.

2 cups broccoli florets

1 cup carrots, sliced in 1/4 inch thick half-moons

1 1/2 cups cooked white beans

1/2 medium purple onion, diced

1/2 red bell pepper, diced

2 tablespoons finely chopped fresh basil

2 tablespoons extra-virgin olive oil

2 tablespoons flaxseed oil

2 tablespoons freshly squeezed lemon juice

1 teaspoon honey mustard

2 teaspoons honey

1/2 teaspoon sea salt, or to taste

fresh-ground black pepper

1. Blanch broccoli and carrots separately in rapidly boiling salted water just until barely tender, approximately 1 minute. Remove and cool under cold running water. Drain.
2. In a large bowl, mix together white beans, purple onion, red bell pepper, and basil. Add broccoli and carrots.
3. Combine olive oil, flaxseed oil, lemon juice, mustard, honey, and sea salt. Pour over bean-and-vegetable mixture. Add freshly ground black pepper and mix gently.
4. Allow to stand for at least 15 minutes before serving, and adjust seasonings.

Citrus Vinaigrette

Fresh orange juice gives this vinaigrette a refreshing, slightly sweet flavor. Flaxseed oil provides beneficial omega-3 oils. This is delicious over mixed leafy greens.

2 tablespoons extra-virgin olive oil

2 tablespoons flaxseed oil

1 tablespoon Dijon mustard

1 tablespoon honey

1/4 teaspoon sea salt, or to taste

1/4 cup freshly squeezed orange juice

1/4 cup freshly squeezed lemon juice

1. Combine olive oil, flaxseed oil, mustard, sea salt, and honey, and mix well.
2. Whisk in orange juice and lemon juice until thoroughly blended, and adjust seasonings.

Creamy Herb-Tofu Dressing

Soft tofu makes a creamy salad dressing and is an easy way to get an extra serving of hormone-balancing phytoestrogens.

2 garlic cloves, minced

1 scallion, white and light-green parts, minced

2 teaspoons freshly squeezed lemon juice

1 tablespoon apple-cider vinegar

1 teaspoon honey

10 ounces soft tofu

1 tablespoon extra-virgin olive oil

1 tablespoon flaxseed oil

1 teaspoon dried oregano

1/2 teaspoon celery seed

sea salt and fresh-ground pepper to taste

Place all ingredients in blender and blend until smooth.

Soups

Miso Soup with Shiitake Mushrooms

Miso is a good source of phytoestrogens and also provides beneficial flora for the intestinal tract. Shiitake mushrooms are potent immune enhancers. Serves 4.

1 tablespoon unhulled sesame seeds

1 tablespoon extra-virgin olive oil

1/2 pound sliced fresh shiitake mushrooms (discard tough stems)

3 cloves garlic, minced

1/4 teaspoon sea salt

5 cups water

2 tablespoons light miso, or to taste

1/4 cup thinly sliced scallions

1. Toast sesame seeds in a large skillet over medium heat until golden. Remove from skillet as soon as they are done to prevent burning.
2. Sauté mushrooms in olive oil for 2 minutes. Add garlic and sea salt and continue sauteeing for an additional 2 minutes. Add vegetable stock or water and simmer gently for 5 minutes. Turn off heat.
3. Dissolve miso in a small amount of hot soup broth and add to soup. Cover, and let stand for 2 minutes.
4. Serve, garnishing each bowl with scallions and sesame seeds.

Carrot-Ginger Soup

This satisfying soup is deliciously rich in the cell-protecting antioxidant beta-carotene. Serves 3–4.

1-1/2 cups onion, chopped

1-1/2 inch fresh ginger root, minced

1/4 teaspoon herb salt or sea salt

2 tablespoons extra-virgin olive oil

4 cups carrots, chopped into 1-inch pieces

1 cup potato, peeled and chopped

1 teaspoon fennel seed

5 cups vegetable or chicken stock (or water)

2 tablespoons light miso (or sea salt to taste)

2 tablespoons minced parsley

1. Sauté onion, ginger, and salt for 2 minutes in olive oil in large soup pot. Add carrots and fennel seed and sauté an additional 3 minutes.
2. Add potato and stock or water and bring to a boil. Cover, reduce heat, and simmer for 20 minutes or until carrots and potato are soft.
3. Turn off heat and puree in small batches with miso in a blender. Return to soup pot and reheat gently if necessary. Serve garnished with finely minced parsley.

Lentil Soup with Roasted Garlic and Kale

Adding dark-leafy greens to bean soup creates a healthful one-dish meal loaded with vitamin K, calcium, and fiber. Serves 4.

> *1 bulb garlic*
>
> *1 cup brown lentils*
>
> *6 cups vegetable or chicken stock (or water)*
>
> *2 sprigs each fresh thyme and oregano*
>
> *1 pound fresh tomatoes, peeled and seeded (or 12 ounces canned tomatoes with juice)*
>
> *2 tablespoons extra-virgin olive oil*
>
> *1/2 teaspoon dried oregano*
>
> *1 teaspoon fennel seed*
>
> *1 teaspoon sea salt (or to taste)*
>
> *1-1/2 cups onion, diced*
>
> *1/2 cup carrot, diced*
>
> *1/2 cup red bell pepper, diced*
>
> *3 cups thinly sliced kale*

1. Rub the head of garlic with a small amount of olive oil and roast on a baking sheet in a preheated 350-degree oven for 30 minutes, or until soft. Remove from oven and allow to cool.

2. Rinse the lentils and place in a soup pot with stock, thyme, and oregano. Bring to a boil, reduce heat, and simmer covered until the lentils are tender, about 20 minutes. Remove the herbs.

3. Slice off the top of the garlic head, and squeeze the garlic out of its skin. Puree the garlic with the tomatoes in a blender, and set aside.

4. Heat the olive oil in a saucepan and sauté the onion, salt, dried oregano, and fennel seed for 3 minutes. Add the carrot and red bell pepper and sauté for an additional 5 minutes. Add the pureed tomato-garlic mixture, and simmer for 10 minutes.

5. Add the sautéed vegetables and kale to the lentils and cook, covered, over low heat for 20 minutes or until kale and lentils are tender. Adjust seasonings, and serve.

Creamy Potato and Kale Soup

Kale and soy milk make potato soup nutrient-rich. Serves 3–4.

> *2 tablespoons extra virgin olive oil*
> *2 cups chopped onion*
> *1 cup chopped celery*
> *1 teaspoon fennel seeds*
> *1 pound potatoes, peeled and diced*
> *1/2 teaspoon sea salt*
> *3 garlic cloves, minced*
> *2 cups vegetable stock or water*
> *1 sprig fresh thyme*
> *2 tablespoons light miso*
> *1 bunch kale, thinly sliced (approximately 6 cups)*
> *3 cups soy milk*

1. Heat olive oil in a heavy soup pot over medium heat and sauté onion, celery, fennel seeds, potatoes, and sea salt for approximately 10 minutes, or until onions are soft. Add garlic and sauté an additional 2 minutes.

2. Add vegetable stock and thyme. Cover, and simmer until potatoes are soft, approximately 10 minutes.

3. Dilute miso in a small amount of hot soup broth and add to pot along with kale. Cook 5 minutes.

4. Add soy milk and cook an additional 5 minutes, taking care not to boil the soup. Adjust seasonings and serve.

Shiitake Mushroom and Barley Soup

This hearty soup contains a hefty dose of immune-enhancing shiitake mushrooms. Serves 4–6.

> *2 tablespoons olive oil*
> *1-1/2 cups diced onion*
> *1/2 teaspoon sea salt*

5 cloves minced garlic

1-1/2-inch piece fresh ginger root, finely chopped

1/2 cup diced carrots

1/2 cup diced celery

5 cups vegetable or chicken stock

1/2 cup dry red wine

1 sprig fresh thyme

1/4 cup pearl barley, rinsed

1 pound shiitake mushrooms, sliced and tough ends discarded

1 teaspoon tamari (natural soy sauce)

1 tablespoon minced fresh parsley

1 teaspoon minced fresh thyme leaves

1. Sauté onion in 1 tablespoon olive oil with sea salt in a soup pot until the onion softens, approximately 5 minutes. Add the garlic, ginger, carrots, and celery, and sauté for an additional 2 minutes.

2. Add 3 cups of the vegetable or chicken stock, wine, thyme, and barley, and simmer, covered, over medium heat until the barley is tender, approximately 30 to 40 minutes.

3. While the soup is cooking, sauté the shiitake mushrooms in two batches, using 1/2 tablespoon of the remaining olive oil and a pinch of sea salt for each batch. Cook over high heat until the mushrooms sear and turn golden. Deglaze the pan with 1/2 cup of the remaining stock and 1/2 teaspoon of tamari, and add the first panful of mushrooms to the soup pot. Repeat the process with the remaining mushrooms, and add to the soup.

4. Simmer all ingredients together for 5 minutes and adjust seasonings. Garnish with minced parsley and thyme leaves.

Dandelion Greens Soup

This refreshing soup is a good way to get the benefits of bitter greens. Serves 4.

1/2 cup onion, diced

1 tablespoon extra-virgin olive oil

1/2 teaspoon fennel seeds

1 pound small new potatoes, cubed

4 cups vegetable broth

1 bunch young dandelion greens, chopped (or watercress)

1/2 bunch parsley, stems removed and chopped

sea salt to taste

1. In a soup pot, sauté onion in olive oil with a pinch of sea salt until translucent, approximately 5 minutes. Add fennel seeds and potatoes and sauté an additional 2 minutes.

2. Add vegetable broth and bring to a boil. Cover the pot, lower the heat, and simmer potatoes until tender, approximately 10 minutes.

3. Add greens and parsley (save some parsley for garnish) and simmer 5 minutes.

4. Puree the soup in several batches in a blender, return to soup pot, and season to taste with sea salt. Garnish with parsley and serve.

Curried Red-Lentil Soup

Lentils are a rich source of soluble fiber, which helps to reduce cholesterol and estrogen levels, and turmeric enhances liver health. Red lentils are especially quick cooking. Serves 4.

1 medium onion, diced

1 inch piece fresh ginger root, sliced thinly

2 tablespoons extra-virgin olive oil

1 teaspoon cumin seeds

1 teaspoon fennel seeds

1 1/2 cups red lentils, washed

4 cups vegetable broth

4 cups water

1 cinnamon stick

1 teaspoon turmeric

3 cups chopped sweet winter squash

2 teaspoons curry powder

1/2 teaspoon sea salt

1/4 cup minced parsley

1. Sauté onion and ginger root with a pinch of sea salt in olive oil for 5 minutes. Add cumin and fennel seeds and sauté for 1 minute.

2. Add lentils, vegetable broth, water, cinnamon, and turmeric, and bring to a boil. Lower heat and simmer for 15 minutes.

3. Add winter squash, curry powder, and sea salt and simmer for an additional 20 minutes.

4. Adjust seasonings, garnish with parsley, and serve.

Entrees

Lemon-Herb Marinated Tofu

This is a simple and delicious way to prepare tofu. It's terrific on sandwiches or in salads. Serves 4.

1 pound firm tofu, drained

Marinade:

2 tablespoons extra-virgin olive oil

1/4 cup tamari (natural soy sauce)

1/2 cup freshly squeezed lemon juice

2 tablespoons balsamic vinegar

2 tablespoons finely chopped fresh rosemary

1 tablespoon crushed fennel seeds

1. Place tofu in a colander for 15 minutes to drain off excess water.

2. Slice tofu into 1-inch thick rectangles and arrange in a single layer in a shallow baking dish.

3. Combine remaining ingredients for marinade and heat in a small saucepan just until the mixture comes to a boil. Pour the marinade over the tofu pieces.

4. Refrigerate for several hours, and preferably overnight. Turn the tofu pieces over at least once to allow them to soak up the marinade evenly.

5. Remove from marinade, and grill tofu on a grill or under the broiler until golden brown.

Marinated Teriyaki Tofu

Marinated tofu makes a great main course with rice and vegetables. If possible, let the tofu marinate for at least several hours, or even better, overnight. Serves 4.

> *1 pound firm tofu, drained*
>
> Marinade:
>
> *2 tablespoons extra-virgin olive oil*
>
> *1 teaspoon toasted sesame oil*
>
> *1/4 cup tamari (natural soy sauce)*
>
> *1/2 cup freshly squeezed orange juice*
>
> *1 tablespoon freshly squeezed lime juice*
>
> *1 tablespoon honey*
>
> *1 tablespoon fresh-grated ginger root*
>
> *2 cloves garlic, minced*
>
> *1/4 teaspoon red pepper flakes*

1. Place tofu in a colander for 15 minutes to drain off excess water.

2. Slice the tofu into 1-inch thick rectangles, and arrange in a single layer in a shallow baking dish.

3. Combine marinade ingredients in a small saucepan and heat just until the mixture comes to a boil. Pour marinade over the tofu pieces.

4. Refrigerate for several hours, and preferably overnight. Turn the tofu pieces over at least once to allow them to soak up the marinade evenly.

5. Remove from marinade and grill tofu on a grill or under the broiler until golden brown.

Scrambled Tofu with Spinach and Shiitake

Rich in phytoestrogens and the health-protective benefits of shiitake, this dish is excellent for breakfast or brunch, or even a light supper. Serves 3–4.

16 ounces extra-firm tofu

4 teaspoons extra-virgin olive oil

1/4 cup finely chopped scallion

1/4 teaspoon turmeric

1/4 teaspoon sea salt

4 ounces shiitake mushrooms, stemmed and thinly sliced

1/2 small bunch spinach, washed and coarsely chopped

1. Drain tofu in a colander for 15 minutes while preparing shiitake and spinach.
2. Heat 2 teaspoons olive oil in a large skillet, and sauté scallions for 1 minute. Crumble tofu into skillet (it should look something like cottage-cheese curds). Add turmeric and sea salt and cook 2 minutes. Remove from skillet.
3. Add remaining 2 teaspoons olive oil to skillet and sauté shiitake with a pinch of sea salt until they release their liquid, about 5 minutes. Add spinach and sauté for an additional 2 minutes until spinach has wilted and liquid has evaporated.
4. Return tofu to skillet and mix with shiitake and spinach. Serve.

Savory Tempeh with Red Peppers

Tempeh makes a satisfying vegetarian entree and is rich in hormone-balancing phytoestrogens. Serves 4.

8 ounces tempeh, sliced into 1/2-inch slices

3 tablespoons tamari (natural soy sauce)

2 tablespoons freshly squeezed orange juice

1 tablespoon freshly squeezed lime juice

1 teaspoon toasted sesame oil

2 tablespoons extra-virgin olive oil

1/2 large red pepper, thinly sliced into 2-inch strips

1/2 medium purple onion, thinly sliced into half-moons

3 garlic cloves, minced

1-inch piece fresh ginger root, minced

1. Mix tamari, orange juice, lime juice, and sesame oil in a large, shallow dish. Add tempeh, and toss to coat with the marinade. Allow to marinate for 30 minutes.

2. Remove tempeh from marinade with slotted spoon, reserving marinade. Heat 1 tablespoon oil in a large nonstick skillet and sauté tempeh. Stir-fry until golden, approximately 3 minutes, and remove tempeh from skillet.

3. Add remaining 1 tablespoon of oil to the skillet and sauté the pepper and onion for about 2 minutes, until they begin to soften. Add the garlic and ginger and continue to sauté for about 3 minutes, until the onions and peppers are cooked.

4. Add the tempeh and marinade, and cook for 2 minutes. Adjust seasonings and serve with rice or pasta and a green vegetable.

Tempeh with Asparagus and Garlic Sauce

This dish provides phytoestrogens from tempeh, glutathione from asparagus, and immune-enhancing garlic. Serves 4.

8 ounces tempeh, sliced lengthwise and then crosswise into 1/4-inch slices

3 tablespoons tamari (natural soy sauce), divided

1 teaspoon freshly squeezed lemon juice

1 cup vegetable broth

3 garlic cloves, minced

1 teaspoon honey mustard

2 tablespoons extra-virgin olive oil, divided

1 pound fresh asparagus, tough stems removed, cut diagonally into 2-inch pieces

1 tablespoon fresh ginger root, grated

1. Combine 1 tablespoon tamari and lemon juice with tempeh in a shallow bowl, and let marinate for 15 minutes.
2. Combine remaining 2 tablespoons tamari with vegetable broth, mustard, and garlic and set aside.
3. Heat 1 tablespoon olive oil in a large, nonstick skillet over medium-high heat and sauté tempeh until golden, about 5 minutes. Be sure to turn the tempeh while sautéing to cook all sides evenly. Remove tempeh from skillet.
4. Add additional tablespoon of olive oil to skillet, and add asparagus and ginger root. Sauté for 1 minute, and add vegetable-broth mixture, cover, and cook for 3 minutes or until asparagus is almost tender.
5. Add tempeh and simmer uncovered for 2–3 minutes uncovered to reduce liquid. Serve over rice or pasta.

Honey-Mustard Glazed Salmon on Mustard Greens

This elegant and delicious dish gives you the double benefit of omega-3 rich salmon and calcium-rich mustard greens. Serves 4.

4 salmon fillets, 6 ounces each

3 tablespoons honey

3 tablespoons Dijon mustard

1 1/2 tablespoons tamari (natural soy sauce)

2 tablespoons freshly squeezed orange juice

1 1/2 teaspoons finely chopped fresh ginger

1 medium garlic clove, minced

fresh-ground black pepper

1 large bunch mustard greens

1. Preheat oven to 425 degrees. Rinse salmon fillets and pat dry. Lightly oil the bottom of an ovenproof baking dish, and arrange the fillets in a single layer in the dish.
2. Mix together honey, mustard, tamari, orange juice, ginger, and garlic. Spread over salmon fillets and add a bit of fresh-ground black pepper. Bake for 15 minutes, or until fish flakes easily with a fork.

3. While fish is cooking, bring 2 cups of water and a pinch of sea salt to boil in a large pot. Wash mustard greens, remove tough stems, and slice into 2-inch-wide strips. Cook mustard greens in boiling water for 3 minutes, or until tender. Drain.

4. To serve, divide mustard greens among four plates, and top with cooked salmon fillets.

Salmon with Red Peppers and Onions

Red peppers and onions add savory sweetness to salmon fillets, and capers add an unexpected zing of flavor. Serves 4.

4 6-ounce salmon fillets

1 tablespoon extra-virgin olive oil

1 large red bell pepper, cut into 1/4-inch strips

1 large purple or yellow onion, thinly sliced

sea salt

2 teaspoons minced fresh oregano (or 1 teaspoon dried)

1 tablespoon balsamic vinegar

1 tablespoon drained capers

fresh oregano sprigs for garnish

1. Preheat oven to 425 degrees. Rinse salmon fillets and pat dry. Lightly oil the bottom of an ovenproof shallow baking dish and arrange the fillets in a single layer.

2. Sauté red pepper and onion in olive oil with a pinch of sea salt and oregano until translucent and tender. Add balsamic vinegar and capers.

3. Spoon vegetables over salmon fillets, and bake for 15 minutes, or until fish flakes easily with a fork. Garnish with oregano sprigs and serve.

Marinated Grilled Salmon

This is an easy, delicious way to prepare omega-3 rich salmon and is great on the grill. Serves 4.

4 6-ounce salmon fillets

Marinade:

1/2 cup tamari (natural soy sauce)

1 cup freshly squeezed orange juice

1 tablespoon freshly squeezed lime juice

1 tablespoon honey

3 cloves garlic, minced

1 tablespoon fresh-grated ginger root

1/4 teaspoon red pepper flakes

1. To make the marinade, mix together all the ingredients except the salmon.
2. Rinse the salmon fillets, and place in a single layer in a shallow glass baking dish. Cover with the marinade and refrigerate for at least 3 hours, turning the fish once while marinating.
3. Drain the fillets and grill or broil until fish flakes with a fork.

Vegetables and Grains

Quick-Cooked Greens

Dark-leafy greens are rich sources of calcium and other minerals. Boiling them quickly in water preserves more nutrients than does steaming, and they taste better. Serves 3–4.

1 bunch kale, collard, or mustard greens

pinch of sea salt

1. Wash greens. Remove tough stems and center ribs and slice greens crosswise into 1-inch-wide strips.
2. Bring 2 cups of water and sea salt to boil in a large pot. Add greens, cover, and cook over high heat for approximately 5 minutes, or until tender. Drain well, add a bit of olive oil or lemon if desired, and serve.

Kale with Pumpkin Seeds and Currants

This is a deliciously, different twist on leafy greens. Kale is rich in beta-carotene and vitamin K, and pumpkin seeds are a good source of essential fatty acids. Serves 4.

1/4 cup pumpkin seeds

1 large bunch kale

1 tablespoon extra-virgin olive oil

1-inch piece of ginger root, peeled and finely chopped

1/4 cup currants

sea salt and lemon

1. Toast pumpkin seeds in a heavy skillet over medium heat, stirring constantly until they turn lightly golden. Remove from skillet to cool.
2. Blanch kale in boiling, salted water for 1 minute. Drain and chop coarsely.
3. Sauté ginger in olive oil in a large, heavy skillet over medium heat for 1 minute, or until golden. Add currants and greens and cook until greens are tender. Season with sea salt and lemon to taste. Add pumpkin seeds and serve.

Sautéed Greens with Garlic and Sesame Seeds

This is a delicious way to eat greens and takes just a few minutes of extra preparation time. Serves 4.

1 tablespoon sesame seeds

1 large bunch greens, such as kale, dandelion, or mustard

1 tablespoon extra-virgin olive oil

2 garlic cloves, minced

sea salt and lemon to taste

1. Toast sesame seeds in a heavy skillet over medium heat for several minutes, stirring constantly until they turn golden. Remove from skillet to cool.

2. Blanch greens quickly in boiling salted water for 1 minute. Drain and chop coarsely.

3. Sauté garlic in olive oil for 30 seconds. Add greens and sea salt and toss to coat with olive oil. Sauté for 2–5 minutes, or until tender.

4. Sprinkle with sesame seeds, add lemon, and adjust seasonings.

Collard Greens with Caramelized Onions

Collard greens are tender and sweet and a good source of carotenes, minerals, and vitamin K. Serves 4.

> *1 tablespoon extra-virgin olive oil*
> *1 onion, thinly sliced into crescents*
> *2 teaspoons balsamic vinegar*
> *1 large bunch collard greens, washed*
> *sea salt*

1. Sauté onions in olive oil over medium heat with a pinch of sea salt until the onions turn golden and very soft (approximately 15–20 minutes). Add balsamic vinegar and cook 3 minutes more.

2. Meanwhile, slice collard greens in half down the middle of the center rib, and then slice crosswise into 1/2-inch pieces.

3. Bring approximately 2 cups of water to boil in a large pot with a pinch of sea salt. Add collard greens and cook, covered, for approximately 5 minutes or until tender. Drain immediately.

4. Add collard greens to onions and mix well. Serve immediately.

Garlic-Chive Mashed Potatoes

These delicious potatoes provide lots of heart-healthy garlic, and are high in fiber if you cook them with the skins. Serves 4.

> *4 cups scrubbed and cubed potatoes (Yukon Gold, Yellow Finn, or red potatoes)*

12 garlic cloves, peeled and chopped

1 tablespoon extra-virgin olive oil

1 tablespoon flaxseed oil

2 tablespoons minced chives

2 tablespoons minced parsley

sea salt and fresh-ground black pepper to taste

1. Place potatoes, garlic, and 1/2 teaspoon sea salt into a pot and add just enough water to barely cover. Bring to a boil, lower the heat, and simmer, covered, for 15 minutes, or until the potatoes are tender. Drain, reserving the cooking liquid.

2. Mash the potatoes and garlic with olive oil and flaxseed oil. Add in reserved cooking liquid, a little at a time, to achieve a fluffy texture.

3. Stir in chives and parsley, and add salt and fresh-ground black pepper to taste.

Asparagus with Garlic and Lemon

Asparagus is rich in the powerful antioxidant glutathione, and garlic strengthens your cardiovascular and immune systems. Serves 4.

1 pound asparagus, tough ends removed

2 tablespoons extra-virgin olive oil

4 large cloves garlic, minced

1 lemon, juiced

sea salt

1. Cook asparagus spears in rapidly boiling salted water until tender, approximately 3–4 minutes. Drain.

2. Meanwhile, heat olive oil in a skillet over medium heat. Add garlic, and sauté for 1 minute, being careful to not burn the garlic. Add the lemon juice, and cook for 1 minute.

3. Toss the olive oil mixture with the asparagus and serve.

Maple Yams with Walnuts

Yams are an exceptionally good source of beta-carotene, and walnuts and flaxseed oil provide a healthy dose of omega-3 essential fatty acids. Serves 4.

4 medium yams

sea salt

2 tablespoons flaxseed oil

4 ounces plain soy milk

1/2 teaspoon ground cinnamon

1 tablespoon maple syrup

2 tablespoons coarsely chopped walnuts

1. Peel yams and slice into 1/2-inch-thick pieces.
2. Place in a large pot, barely cover with water, add a pinch of sea salt, and bring to a boil. Reduce cover, heat and simmer until soft. Drain.
3. Place yams in a large bowl and mash. Add flaxseed oil, soy milk, cinnamon, and maple syrup and blend well.
4. Garnish with walnuts and serve.

Quinoa with Fresh Corn and Red Peppers

Quinoa is a quick-cooking mineral-rich grain that makes a fluffy pilaf. This is a terrific side dish with fish, chicken, or tofu, or tempeh. Serves 4.

1 cup quinoa

1 tablespoon extra-virgin olive oil

1/2 cup purple onion, finely chopped

1/2 cup red bell pepper, finely chopped

2 cloves garlic, minced

2 cups vegetable stock or water

1 cup fresh corn kernels

1/2 teaspoon sea salt

1/4 cup fresh parsley, minced

1. Rinse quinoa in a fine-mesh strainer and drain.
2. In a heavy pot over medium heat, sauté onion and red bell pepper in olive oil for 2 minutes. Add garlic, and sauté 1 minute. Add quinoa and vegetable stock, corn, and sea salt. Bring to a boil, cover, reduce heat, and simmer for 15 minutes.
3. Turn off heat and add parsley. Let sit, covered, for 5 minutes. Fluff quinoa with a fork and serve.

Wild Rice Pilaf

Wild rice is rich in minerals and fiber and has a delicious nutty flavor. Serves 4.

1 tablespoon extra-virgin olive oil

1/2 cup onion, finely chopped

1/2 cup red bell pepper, finely chopped

sea salt

1/2 cup wild rice

3/4 cup brown basmati rice

1 1/2 cups vegetable or chicken stock

1 cup water

2 tablespoons pine nuts, lightly toasted

2 tablespoons parsley, finely minced

1. Sauté onion and red pepper with a pinch of sea salt in olive oil in a heavy, medium-sized pot for 3 minutes.
2. Add the wild and brown rice and sauté for 2 minutes, then add the broth and water and 1/4 teaspoon sea salt.
3. Bring to a simmer, lower the heat, and cover. Let simmer for 55 minutes, turn off the heat, and allow to stand, covered, for an additional 5 minutes.
4. Fluff with a fork, garnish with pine nuts and parsley, and serve.

Fruit Beverages and Desserts

Mixed-Berry Yogurt Smoothie

This smoothie makes a delicious purple shake. The berries provide an excellent source of cell-protective nutrients, and yogurt adds calcium. Serves 2.

> *1 cup frozen blueberries*
> *1/2 cup frozen raspberries*
> *1 medium banana, peeled and cut into 1-inch chunks*
> *12 ounces plain yogurt*
> *1/2 teaspoon vanilla extract*
> *1 teaspoon maple syrup, if desired*

Combine all ingredients in blender and blend until smooth.

Strawberry-Citrus Smoothie

This smoothie is a refreshing way to start the day. Strawberries, peaches, and orange juice are high in vitamin C. Serves 2.

> *1 1/2 cups freshly squeezed orange juice*
> *1 cup frozen strawberries*
> *1 cup fresh peaches, peeled and diced*
> *1 medium banana, peeled and cut into 1-inch chunks*

Combine all ingredients in blender, and blend until smooth.

Banana-Almond Smoothie

This satisfying smoothie tastes almost like a milk shake if you use frozen bananas. Cut bananas into 1-inch chunks and freeze on a cookie sheet, then store in a plastic container in the freezer for up to 1 month. If you are not using frozen bananas, add several ice cubes to the smoothie. Almonds and yogurt provide a healthful dose of calcium. Serves 2.

12 ounces plain yogurt

2 medium bananas, cut into 1-inch chunks and frozen

2 tablespoons chopped almonds

1/2 teaspoon vanilla extract

Combine all ingredients in blender and blend until smooth.

Raspberry-Soy Smoothie

This flavorful drink makes a good breakfast beverage or snack that is rich in vitamin C and health-protective phytoestrogens. Serves 1.

1 medium banana, peeled and cut into chunks

1 cup plain soy milk

1 tablespoon frozen orange-juice concentrate

1/2 cup frozen strawberries

1/2 cup frozen raspberries

1. Blend banana, soy milk and orange juice concentrate in blender until mixed.
2. Add frozen strawberries and raspberries, and blend until smooth and creamy.

Exotic Fruit Salad with Citrus Dressing

This combination of fruits supplies abundant amounts of antioxidants and health-protective phytochemicals. Serves 4.

2 large, ripe mangoes, peeled, pitted, and diced

4 kiwi fruit, peeled and sliced

2 cups stemmed and sliced strawberries

2 cups blueberries

1/4 cup fresh orange juice

1 tablespoon fresh lime juice

1 tablespoon honey

1 tablespoon julienned crystallized ginger

1. Combine fruit in a large serving bowl.
2. Mix together orange juice, lime juice, and honey. Drizzle over fruit and toss gently to combine.
3. Garnish with crystallized ginger and serve.

Gingered Fruit Compote

This compote has gentle laxative properties and is excellent with yogurt. Yields 4 cups.

> *1 pound assorted dried prunes, currants, apricots, and apples*
> *1 stick cinnamon*
> *1-inch piece fresh ginger root, sliced thinly*
> *pinch sea salt*

1. Place ingredients in a heavy saucepan and add enough water to just cover the fruit.
2. Simmer, covered, over low heat for 1 hour, stirring occasionally.
3. Keep refrigerated for up to 1 week.

Peaches in Raspberry-Strawberry Sauce

Peaches, strawberries, and raspberries are good sources of vitamin C, and strawberries and raspberries contain ellagic acid, a cancer-preventive nutrient. Serves 4.

> *4 large ripe peaches, sliced*
> *1/2 pint strawberries, washed, hulled, and sliced*
> *1/2 pint raspberries, washed*
> *1 tablespoon maple syrup*
> *2 tablespoon almonds, lightly toasted and chopped*
> *fresh mint leaves*

1. Purée strawberries and raspberries in blender with maple syrup.
2. Arrange peaches on dessert plates, and pour the fruit sauce over the peaches. Garnish with toasted almonds and fresh mint leaves.

Apples Poached with Cinnamon, Nutmeg, and Vanilla

Apples are rich in pectin, a soluble fiber. This makes a delicious breakfast accompaniment or dessert. Serves 4.

4 cups apple juice

2 cinnamon sticks

1/8 teaspoon ground nutmeg

1/2 vanilla bean

4 firm apples

2 fresh mint leaves

1. Combine apple juice, cinnamon sticks, nutmeg, and vanilla bean in a pot large enough to hold apples in a single layer.
2. Peel and core apples and add to liquid. Add additional apple juice if necessary to cover the apples. Bring to a simmer over medium heat, and cook gently just until apples are tender, approximately 10 minutes.
3. Remove apples from liquid and place in a large bowl. Remove cinnamon sticks and vanilla bean and reduce poaching liquid to a syrup by simmering uncovered for approximately 30 minutes.
4. Pour over apples and cool to room temperature. Chill before serving.
5. To serve, place apples in dessert bowls and spoon syrup over apples. Garnish with fresh mint leaves.

Appendix II

Natural Healing Treatments

There are many natural, simple methods for enhancing your health and well-being that you can easily practice at home. Some of these, such as relaxation exercises and meditation, are practices that you may want to incorporate into your everyday life. Others, such as sitz baths and compresses, are meant to be used as treatments for specific health conditions.

Breathing Exercises

Your breath is one of the most powerful tools you have for relaxing your body and mind, building vitality, and improving your health. Your breath connects your mind and body, and when you consciously focus your attention on your breathing, you immediately and positively influence your physical and emotional well-being. Learning to breathe fully in a relaxed way is one of the quickest ways to energize and heal your body and calm your mind, but it often takes conscious practice to transform old breathing habits that cause fatigue and tension into new, healthier ways of breathing. Set aside 5 or 10 minutes every day to practice one or more of the following breathing exercises. When you become familiar with conscious breathing techniques, you can practice them anywhere, at any time. If you've never before practiced deep breathing exercises, you might initially find that you feel a bit lightheaded. Go slowly with the exercises, and work at a pace that feels comfortable to you.

Simple Relaxing Breath

This easy exercise slows down your breathing and helps you to feel calm, relaxed, and energized.

- Sit in a comfortable position with your back straight, and bring your attention to your breathing.
- Relax, and inhale through your nose to a count of 5, counting at a pace that is comfortable for you.
- Hold your breath for a count of 5.
- Open your mouth slightly, and exhale to a count of 10, keeping your exhalation smooth and controlled.
- Repeat the exercise for a total of five complete cycles.

Deep Belly Breathing

Deep belly breathing (also called diaphragmatic or abdominal breathing) teaches you to breathe correctly. Observe a young child, and you'll get the idea of how you should breathe. When you inhale, your abdomen should expand, and when you exhale, your abdomen should contract. This is just the opposite of how most adults breathe. Chronic stress and internalizing messages such as "hold in your stomach" lead to poor breathing habits. To restore a healthy breathing pattern, practice the following exercise.

- Lie on your back with your knees bent and your feet flat on the floor about hip-width apart, a comfortable distance from your buttocks. Place your hands on your abdomen to help you feel the expansion and contraction of your abdomen as you breathe.

- Inhale slowly and deeply, allowing your breath to fill and expand your abdomen. As you inhale, gently arch your lower back, which helps to expand your abdomen and relaxes your internal organs.
- Exhale, gently pulling your abdominal muscles in toward your spine, at the same time gently flattening the small of your back against the floor.
- Continue breathing in this way for several minutes, and then relax.

Alternate Nostril Breathing

This yoga breathing exercise calms the body and mind and promotes clear thinking by balancing the right and left hemispheres of the brain.

- Sit in a comfortable position with your spine straight and your shoulders relaxed.
- Gently press your right nostril closed with your right thumb and inhale slowly and deeply to a count of 5 through your left nostril. Gently press your left nostril closed with the ring finger of your right hand. Retain the breath for a count of 5.
- Release your thumb, exhaling slowly and completely through your right nostril to a count of 10. Immediately inhale through your right nostril in a slow and steady rhythm to a count of 5. Close your right nostril with your right thumb and retain the breath for count of 5.
- Release your ring finger, and exhale slowly and steadily through your left nostril to a count of 10. Repeat the entire sequence five to ten times, keeping your breath even and controlled.

Vitality-Enhancing Breath

This simple breathing exercise provides a boost of quick energy.

- Sit or stand with your spine straight and your shoulders relaxed.
- Inhale a series of short, quick breaths through your nostrils until your lungs are completely filled with air.

- Exhale forcefully and quickly through your mouth, making the sound "ha" as you exhale completely.
- Repeat several times, and then resume normal breathing.

Relaxation and Visualization Exercises

Relaxation exercises help you to recognize and release tension that you hold in your body. Stressful patterns of behavior are learned responses, and the best way to change them is to set aside time to consciously practice the art of relaxation. Relaxation exercises are beneficial for virtually any physical ailment—from headaches to hypertension—because deep relaxation encourages the free flow of energy and helps to bring your body into a state of balance. Deep relaxation also helps to calm your mind and brings about a sense of peace and well-being.

Visualization takes relaxation a step further, as it channels the power of your imagination to evoke changes in your mind and body. When you create a mental image of what you would like to manifest, your body and mind respond to the picture as though it were a real experience. When practiced on a regular basis, visualization can improve your health and can help you to replace negative habits with positive, life-affirming ones.

You might find it helpful to tape the following exercises or to have a friend read them to you so that you can fully appreciate the experience.

Gentle Progressive Relaxation

This exercise helps you to identify the way that you hold tension in your body through first tensing and then relaxing your muscles. When you tense a muscle, do it gently—just enough to help you focus your attention on that muscle.

Lie down in a comfortable position and close your eyes. Take a deep, easy breath, expanding your abdomen as you inhale. Exhale completely, allowing your abdomen to naturally sink toward your spine. Take a couple of easy breaths in this way, and focus on the rhythm of your breath as it enters and leaves your body. As you exhale, imagine that you are exhaling worries and tension with your breath. Release all of your concerns as you take this time for deep, healing relaxation.

Consciously focus your attention on your feet. Feel the air around your feet, the surface that your feet are resting upon, and become aware of any tension you are holding in your feet. Gently curl your toes as you inhale, hold your inhalation for a moment, and with your next exhalation, relax your feet and toes.

Move your attention to your lower legs, becoming aware of any tension in your calves. Inhale, gently tense your calves, hold your inhalation for a moment, and as you exhale, relax your calves and feel the tension flowing out of your lower legs and down through your feet. Bring your attention to your upper legs and notice any tension that you are holding in your thighs. Inhale while gently tensing your thigh muscles, hold your inhalation for a moment, and then as you exhale, relax your thighs. Take another deep, easy breath, and feel the tension flowing out of your thighs, down your calves, and out of your feet as you exhale.

Become aware of your hips and buttocks resting against the surface on which you are lying. Notice any tension that you are holding in your hips, and as you inhale, gently tense your buttocks muscles. Hold the tension for a moment, and as you exhale, relax your buttocks and hips. Move your attention to your lower back, and become aware of tension that you are holding there. Inhale deeply as you gently arch your lower back, hold the inhalation for a moment, and then relax as you release the tension from your lower back. Take another deep, relaxing breath, and let any remaining tension in your lower back, hips, buttocks, thighs, and calves flow down your legs and out of your feet with your exhalation. Notice and enjoy the feeling of deep relaxation that comes with the release of tension.

Move your attention to your shoulders, and become aware of tension that you are holding there. Inhale, and gently tense your shoulder muscles by raising your shoulders toward your ears. Hold the tension for a moment, and then release it as you exhale. Focus your attention on your upper arms and gently contract the muscles of your upper arms as you inhale. Hold the contraction, and then relax and let go of the tension with your exhalation. Notice any tension in your lower arms and hands, inhale, and gently curl your fists into balls and tighten the muscles in your forearms. Hold the contraction for a moment, and then release it as you exhale. Expand your attention to include your shoulders, upper arms, lower arms, and hands, being aware of any remaining tension. Take a deep, relaxing breath, and as you exhale, let go of any lingering tension, allowing it to flow down your arms and out of your hands.

Bring your attention to your upper back, neck, and head, and notice the surface upon which your head and upper back are resting. Become aware of any tension that you are holding in your head, neck, and upper back. Contract these muscles as you inhale, and hold the contraction for a moment. With a deep exhalation, let the tension flow out of your upper back, neck, and head. Take another deep, relaxing breath, and let go of any residual tension. Notice any tightness in your forehead and around your eyes, and gently tense these muscles as you inhale. Hold the tension for a moment, and then release it as you exhale. Let your attention move to your mouth and jaw, and as you inhale, simply notice any tension here without clenching your jaw. As you exhale, allow your jaw to drop slightly, and relax your mouth and jaw completely. Take another deep inhalation and hold it for a moment. As you exhale, release any remaining tension in your scalp, face, head, and neck, and allow it to flow down through your shoulders, your arms, and out of your hands and fingers.

Move your attention to your chest, and notice the subtle movement of your chest as you inhale. Take a deep inhalation, expand your chest by gently arching your upper back, and hold the inhalation for a moment. Exhale, and let tension flow out of your chest, down your arms, and out through your fingertips. Let your attention move to your abdomen, and notice how your abdomen expands as you inhale. Inhale deeply, expanding your abdomen fully, and hold the inhalation for a moment. Exhale, and let go of any tightness in your abdominal area.

Inhale a deep, easy breath, and imagine your breath filling your entire body with healing relaxation. As you exhale, visualize any remaining tension flowing out of your body. Continue breathing in a relaxed and easy manner for a few minutes, enjoying the deep sense of peace and relaxation that comes from letting go of tension. When you are ready, inhale deeply, stretch, and gently open your eyes as you return to a state of full alertness.

Healing Visualization

This visualization begins with a deep relaxation that prepares your mind and body to receive the healing images you create. You can use this exercise to improve your overall well-being, or to focus on a specific health concern.

Lie in a comfortable position with your eyes closed. Take a deep, easy breath and begin to relax your body and your mind. Focus your attention on your breath, noticing the rising and falling of your abdomen as your breath enters and leaves your body. Without effort, scan your body for tension. Breathe into any tightness that you find and release it with your exhalation. Take three deep, easy breaths, allowing your body and mind to become more deeply relaxed with each exhalation.

Now imagine in your mind's eye a blank screen. Inhale, and visualize the number 5 on the screen. See the number 5 clearly in your mind. As you exhale, visualize the number 5 slowly fading. Take a deep, relaxing inhalation, and see the number 4 appear on the screen in your mind. Exhale, and allow the number 4 to gradually fade. As you inhale again, see the number 3 appear on the screen. Notice how relaxed you are feeling as you exhale, and watch the number 3 slowly fade. Inhale, and visualize the number 2 on the screen. Exhale, watching the number 2 fade, and allow yourself to become even more deeply relaxed. Inhale, and see the number 1 appear on the screen. As you exhale completely, watch the number 1 fade, leaving the screen blank.

Patiently watch the screen in your mind's eye as an image begins to appear. See yourself on the screen, lying comfortably in a beautiful meadow. It is a warm, sunny day, and you are completely safe and protected. Feel the warmth of the sunlight on your body and the gentle breeze caressing your skin. See the rich green of the velvety grass, the deep azure blue of the sky, and the white puffy clouds drifting above you. Smell the sweet freshness of the meadow grasses and flowers, and hear the pleasing sounds of the rustle of leaves in the warm breeze, the faint chirping of birds in the trees, and the melodious bubbling of a gentle nearby stream. Allow yourself to sink even more deeply into this peaceful place, knowing that you are safe and protected. You are warm, comfortable, and completely safe.

Feel the warmth of the sun, and as you inhale, imagine that your body is filled with the golden healing light of the sun's rays. Imagine every cell and organ of your body being bathed, purified, and healed by this warm, soothing light. Notice any place where the energy seems to get stuck, and breathe into that place, using your breath and the purifying light to gently dissolve the blockage. Allow the healing energy of the golden light to flow freely throughout your body. Take a few minutes to scan your entire body while you inhale healing, soothing, golden light and exhale tension. Visualize your organs working in perfect harmony, and see yourself in vibrant health. Acknowledge the deep relaxation and health that you are experiencing, and know that you can access this state of well-being at any time. Relax in this place of balance for a few minutes, enjoying the feeling of being in perfect health.

When you are ready, take a deep breath, and begin to slowly bring your attention back to the present moment. Become aware of your surroundings, stretch your arms and legs, and gently open your eyes while maintaining a feeling of deep calmness and well-being.

Meditation Exercises

Meditation has been practiced for centuries in many spiritual traditions as a way of bringing the body, mind, and spirit into harmonious balance. Basically, meditation involves quieting the mind, which helps you to know yourself in a deeper way. This can help you become aware of habitual patterns of thinking and enable you to make better choices about how you are living. Many people find that meditation is an excellent way of relieving stress, because when the mind is calm, the body naturally follows.

For all forms of meditation, there are a few guidelines that will help to make your experience more beneficial. First, find a quiet place where you will not be disturbed, and choose a time when your stomach is empty, or at least one hour after a meal. Many people find early morning to be a beneficial time for meditation. If you are sitting on a chair, place your feet flat on the floor and sit upright, away from the back of the chair. You can place a firm pillow behind your lower back for support if you wish. If you are sitting on the floor, sit on the edge of a firm cushion to help to keep your spine erect, and cross your legs in a comfortable position.

Rest your hands comfortably on your thighs or in your lap. Gently close your eyes to help to focus your attention inward. Begin each meditation practice with a couple of deep cleansing breaths to release tension from your body. Plan to meditate for 15 to 30 minutes at a time, and establish a regular time and place for your meditation practice. You will enjoy the greatest benefits from meditation when you make it a regular part of your daily life.

Meditation on the Breath

By centering your attention on your breath, your mind and body relax into a peaceful, harmonious state of balance.

Find a quiet place where you will not be disturbed and sit in a comfortable position. Close your eyes, and begin by taking three deep, easy breaths to relax your body, exhaling slowly and completely through your slightly open mouth. Relax into your normal breathing pattern, inhaling and exhaling through your nose.

Focus your attention in a gentle way on your breathing. Simply observe your breathing, without trying to change it in any way. As a point of focus, it can be helpful to center your attention on the rising and falling of your abdomen or on your breath as it enters and exits through your nostrils. When your attention wanders, gently bring your focus back to your breath. With practice, your breathing will fall into an easy, natural rhythm. Continue in this way for 15 to 30 minutes. When you are finished with your meditation, expand your attention to include your surroundings, and gently open your eyes.

Meditation on a Mantra

A mantra is a word or phrase that you silently recite over and over to give your mind a peaceful focus. Choose a word or phrase that has meaning for you. It can be as simple as "peace" or "I am calm."

Sit in a comfortable position, close your eyes, and take three slow, deep breaths, making your exhalation twice as long as your inhalation. Focus your attention on your mantra, and recite the word over and over in your mind. Breathe normally, and synchronize your mantra with your breathing by repeating it on each exhalation. When your mind wanders, gently bring your attention back to your mantra. Continue your mantra meditation for 15 to 30 minutes. At the end of your meditation, sit quietly for a couple of minutes, expand your attention to include your surroundings, and then gently open your eyes.

Once you have chosen a mantra and feel satisfied with it, stick with it. The word will become associated with the feelings of peace and well-being that you experience during meditation, and you will be able to elicit a deep sense of calmness at any time by recalling your mantra.

Journal Writing

Many times, women know that they are anxious, depressed, or unhappy, but are unable to identify the cause of their unhappiness or are uncertain as to how to make changes that will result in a more satisfying life. Unexpressed or unacknowledged feelings are almost always at the root of emotional pain. Journal writing is a simple, yet extremely powerful tool for dissolving emotional blocks and for cultivating self-understanding. Even if you are not feeling emotionally stuck, journal writing is a wonderful tool for accessing your inner wisdom. Studies have shown that people who engage in journal writing on a regular basis enhance the functioning of their immune systems and are less prone to illness.

While you don't have to adhere to a schedule to benefit from journal writing, it does help to set aside time on a regular basis for journaling. You may find that you enjoy writing in the early morning hours, when your mind is fresh and you can still access insights and images from your dreams. Or, you may find that you like to journal just before sleeping as a way of processing the day's events. When you are writing, don't worry about grammar or punctuation—you'll more readily access feelings if you bypass your intellect. Simply allow the free flow of thoughts and images that appear in your mind to be transferred directly to the paper by your hand. It may take a few journal sessions to feel relaxed about writing in this way, but you'll soon discover the unique insights into the inner workings of your mind that appear when you allow your thoughts to flow freely onto the paper. As you continue in your process of journal writing, you will strengthen your connection to your inner wisdom, which will help to guide you toward a healthy, fulfilling, and joyful life.

Hydrotherapy

From the beginning of civilization, water has been revered as an important healing therapy in cultures around the world. Hydrotherapy treatments are based on the use of water in all of its forms—hot and cold water, ice, and steam—to stimulate healing. Hydrotherapy can be used to increase circulation and lymphatic flow, ease pain, and relieve muscular tension. Forms of hydrotherapy that you can easily use at home include sitz baths, foot baths, and compresses.

Sitz Baths

Sitz baths alleviate congestion in the abdominal organs and stimulate circulation and lymphatic flow in the pelvic region. They take a bit of effort, but are an effective treatment for menstrual cramps, cystitis, and fibroids. Use sitz baths as often as desired, or at least every other day when treating a chronic condition such as uterine fibroids.

- You'll need two plastic tubs that are large enough to comfortably hold your buttocks. The purpose of this treatment is to focus the hot and cold baths on your pelvic region to stimulate circulation, so the water should reach only to your navel, leaving your upper body, legs, and feet out of the water.

- Fill one tub with water as hot as you can tolerate. Fill the other tub with ice cold water. You'll only need to fill the tub halfway or less with water—you'll be able to determine how much water you need by sitting in the tub. It usually takes a bit of experimentation to get the amount of water and the temperature just right. The hot tub should be approximately 105-110 degrees F, and the cold tub should be between 55-65 degrees F. You may need to add ice cubes to the cold tub to obtain the desired temperature. Add 7 drops of essential oil to the hot bath, mixing the oil into the water with your hand. Use lavender or marjoram for menstrual cramps; sandalwood or juniper for cystitis; and ginger for uterine fibroids.

- Begin by lowering your buttocks into the hot tub—the water will feel uncomfortably hot at first. Sit with your upper body and legs out of the tub, and make sure that your pelvic region is covered up to your navel with the water. Stay in the hot water for three minutes, and then immediately move to the cold tub for one minute.

- Alternate between the hot and cold tubs three times, remaining in the hot tub each time for three minutes and the cold tub for one minute. Finish with the cold tub, towel off briskly, and rest for a few minutes, focusing your attention on the healing flow of energy circulating throughout your pelvis.

Lymph-Stimulating Foot Bath

Alternating hot and cold foot baths help to stimulate lymphatic flow and also relieve tired, aching feet and legs. They are especially helpful for varicose veins. Use these foot baths as often as desired.

- You'll need two buckets large enough to hold both of your feet, and ideally deep enough so that the water will reach to the middle of your calves to help to stimulate lymphatic flow.
- Fill one bucket with water as hot as you can tolerate (approximately 105-110 degrees F). Fill the other bucket with ice cold water (approximately 55-65 degrees F—you may need to add ice cubes to obtain the desired temperature). Add 7 drops of rosemary essential oil to the bucket of hot water to further stimulate circulation.
- Sit in a comfortable chair and immerse both of your feet in the hot water for three minutes. Immediately plunge your feet into the bucket of cold water for one minute. Repeat the cycle three to five times, ending with the cold water plunge.

Ginger Compress

Hot ginger compresses stimulate increased circulation and are helpful for treating uterine fibroids and menstrual cramps. Use ginger compresses as needed for easing menstrual cramps, and at least every other day for uterine fibroids.

- Grate a handful of fresh ginger root, place in a piece of cheesecloth, twist to make a ball, and tie with a piece of string.

- Fill a large pot with one gallon of water, squeeze the juice from the ginger into the water, and drop the ball of ginger into the water. Cover the pot and heat the water, but do not boil it.

- Turn off the heat. Make a compress by folding a cotton hand-towel in half lengthwise. Dip the towel into the hot ginger water, keeping the ends dry to prevent burning your fingers.

- Wring the compress out and place it over your abdomen, being careful to not burn your skin. You might need to let the compress cool for a few seconds before placing it onto your skin.

- Cover the compress with a thick, dry towel to retain the heat. When the hot towel cools to body temperature, replace it with a fresh hot compress.

- Continue placing hot compresses over your abdomen until your skin turns bright red, which usually takes about 15 to 20 minutes.

Resources

Alternative Health Practitioners

American Association of Oriental Medicine
433 Front Street
Catasauqua, PA 18032
(888) 500-7999

American Association of Naturopathic Physicians
2366 Eastlake Avenue, Suite 322
Seattle, WA 98102
(206) 323-7610

American Holistic Medical Association
6728 Old McLean Village Drive
McLean, VA 22101
(703) 556-9728

Ayurvedic Institute
11311 Menaul N.E., Suite A
Albuquerque, NM 87112
(505) 291-9698

Aromatherapy

The National Association of Holistic Aromatherapists
1-888-275-6242

RECOMMENDED READING:

The Encyclopedia of Essential Oils, by Julia Lawless (Element, 1992)

Aromatherapy: A Complete Guide to the Healing Art, by Kathi Keville and Mindy Green
(The Crossing Press, 1995)

MAIL-ORDER ESSENTIAL OILS:

Prima Fleur Botanicals
1525 East Francisco Boulevard Suite 16
San Rafael, CA 94901
(415) 455-0957

Simpler's Botanical Co.
P. O. Box 2534
Sebastapol, CA 95473
(800) 652-7646

Herbs

INFORMATION AND REFERRALS:

American Botanical Council
6200 Manor Road
Austin, TX 78723
(800) 373-7105

American Herb Association
P. O. Box 1673
Nevada City, CA 95959
(530) 265-9552

Herb Research Foundation
1007 Pearl Street, Suite 200
Boulder, CO 80302
(303) 449-2265

RECOMMENDED READING:

General Herbal:

Herbs for Health and Healing, by Kathi Keville (Rodale Press, 1996)
The Complete Illustrated Holistic Herbal, by David Hoffmann (Element, 1996)
The Green Pharmacy, by James Duke (Rodale Press, 1997)

Women's Herbal:

Herbal Healing for Women, by Rosemary Gladstar (Fireside, 1993)
Herbal Remedies for Women, by Amanda McQuade Crawford (Prima Publishing, 1997)
Menopausal Years The Wise Woman Way, by Susun Weed (Ash Tree Publishing, 1992)
Women's Herbs, Women's Health, by Christopher Hobbs and Kathi Keville (Botanica
     Press, 1998)

Chinese Herbal:

Between Heaven and Earth, A Guide to Chinese Medicine, by Harriet Beinfield and
     Efrem Korngold (Ballantine Books, 1991)

Plant Identification:

Identifying and Harvesting Edible and Medicinal Plants, by Steve Brill (Hearst Books,
     1994)

MAIL-ORDER HERBS:

Avena Botanicals
219 Mill St.
Rockport, ME 04856
(207) 594-0694
herbs, extracts, salves, bodycare

Herb Pharm
Box 116
Williams, OR 97544
(800) 348-4372
extracts, salves

Mountain Rose Herbs
P. O. Box 2000
Redway, CA 95560
(800) 879-3337
herbs, extracts, salves, bodycare

Wise Woman Herbals
P. O. Box 279
Creswell, OR 97426
(541) 895-5172
extracts, salves

MAIL-ORDER CHINESE HERBS:

East Earth Trade Winds
P. O. Box 493151
Redding, CA 96049
(800) 258-6878

Massage

RECOMMENDED BOOKS AND VIDEO:

The Book of Massage, by Lucinda Lidell (Fireside, 1984)
The Book of Shiatsu, by Paul Lundberg (Fireside, 1992)
Massage for Health (Healing Arts video, available from Living Arts catalogue: see *Yoga)*

Natural Bodycare Products

RECOMMENDED READING:

The Herbal Body Book, by Stephanie Tourles (Storey Publishing, 1994)
The Essential Oils Book, by Colleen Dodt (Storey Publishing, 1996)

MAIL-ORDER RESOURCES:

See catalogues listed under *Herbs, Natural Lifestyle,* and *Vitamins*

Natural Lifestyle and Home

RECOMMENDED READING:

Nontoxic, Natural, and Earthwise, by Debra Lynn Dadd (Tarcher, 1990)

MAIL-ORDER CATALOGUE:

Harmony
360 Interlocken Boulevard, Suite 300
Broomfield, CO 80021
(800) 456-1177

Natural Healing

RECOMMENDED READING:

Natural Health magazine
For subscription information:
P.O. Box 37474
Boone, IA 50037
(800) 526-8440

Encyclopedia of Natural Medicine, by Michael Murray, N.D. and Joseph Pizzorno, N.D.
    (Prima Publishing, 1998)

Women's Bodies, Women's Wisdom, by Christiane Northrup, M.D. (Bantam Books, 1998)

8 Weeks to Optimum Health, by Andrew Weil, M.D. (Knopf, 1997)

*14-Day Herbal Cleansing: A Step-by-Step Guide to All Natural Inner Cleansing Techniques
    for Increased Energy, Vitality, and Beauty,* by Laurel Vukovic (Prentice Hall, 1998)

Organic Foods

Diamond Organics
Freedom, CA 95019
(888) 674-2642
mail-order fresh fruits and vegetables

Natural Lifestyles Supplies
16 Lookout Drive
Asheville, NC 28804
(828) 254-9606

Relaxation, Meditation, and Breathwork

RECOMMENDED READING:

Conscious Breathing: Breathwork for Health, Stress Release, and Personal Mastery, by
    Gay Hendricks, Ph.D. (Bantam Books, 1995)

Wherever You Go, There You Are: Mindfulness Meditation in Everyday Life, by Jon Kabat-
    Zinn (Hyperion, 1994)

Vitamins and Supplements

The Vitamin Shoppe
4700 Westside Avenue
North Bergen, New Jersey 07047
(800) 223-1216
mail-order supplements, herbs, and bodycare products

Yoga

RECOMMENDED VIDEOS:

Yoga Journal's Yoga Practice Series
Embracing Menopause, with Susan Winter Ward

Both available from Living Arts catalogue
(800) 254-8464

Index

A

Adrenal depletion, and menopause, 82
Aerobic exercise, 279
    and cancer, 256
    and fibroids, 56
    and menopause, 87
Age spots, 275
Aging gracefully, keys to, 2-3
Aging skin, common signs of, 275
Agni, 198
Alcohol:
    and cancer, 257
    and fatigue, 112-13
    and hypertension, 236, 237
Allium family, and cancer, 252
Alpha-hydroxy acids, 278
Aloe-Lavender Facial Mist, 287-88, 289
Ama, 198
American ginseng:
    and osteoporosis, 213
    and sexual vitality, 103
    and stress, 129-30
Androgens, 81
Anemia, and fatigue, 114
Anise seeds, and hot flashes, 89-90
Antioxidants, 230
    and cancer, 255-56
    and cardiovascular health, 216-17
Anxiety, 124-26
    journaling to relieve, 135-36
    talking to relieve, 135-36
    See also Stress
Apple-cider vinegar, and vaginal infections, 51

Apples, and cancer, 253
Apples Poached with Cinnamon, Nutmeg, and Vanilla, 323
Aromatherapy Body Oil, 295-96
Aromatherapy Compress for Migraine Headaches, 190
Aromatherapy Compress for Tension Headaches, 190
Aromatherapy Facial Mask, 284
Aromatherapy Facial Mist, 287
Aromatherapy Facial Oil, 288
Aromatherapy Facial Sauna, 282, 289
Aromatherapy Nail Oil, 293, 294
Aromatherapy Shampoo, 291-92
    for dry hair, 291
    for hair loss, 292
    for normal hair, 292
    for oily hair, 291
    for problem scalps, 292
Aromatherapy treatments, 4
    for cramps, 31-32
    for depression, 145-46
    for fibroids, 59
    for headaches, 189-90
    for hot flashes, 90
    for hypertension, 241-42
    for memory, 164
    for PMS, 21-22
    for sleep disturbances, 155-56
    for stress, 133-35
    for urinary tract infections (UTIs), 41-42
    for vaginal infections, 50
    for varicose veins, 182-83
Art of conscious living, cultivating, 137-38